£93.99

ONCOPLASTIC
SURGERY OF THE BREAST

ONCOPLASTIC SURGERY OF THE BREAST

MAURICE Y NAHABEDIAN MD FACS

ASSOCIATE PROFESSOR OF PLASTIC SURGERY
DEPARTMENT OF PLASTIC SURGERY
GEORGETOWN UNIVERSITY HOSPITAL
WASHINGTON, DC USA

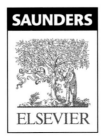

SAUNDERS

ELSEVIER

SAUNDERS
ELSEVIER

an imprint of Elsevier Limited

ISBN: 978-0-7020-3181-6

British Library Cataloguing in Publication Data
Nahabedian, Maurice
  Oncoplastic surgery of the breast
  1. Mammaplasty 2. Breast – Cancer – Patients – Rehabilitation
  I. Title
  618.1'90592

  ISBN-13: 9780702031816

Library of Congress Cataloging in Publication Data
A catalog record for this book is available from the Library of Congress

Notice

Medical knowledge is constantly changing. Standard safety precautions must be followed, but as new research and clinical experience broaden our knowledge, changes in treatment and drug therapy may become necessary or appropriate. Readers are advised to check the most current product information provided by the manufacturer of each drug to be administered to verify the recommended dose, the method and duration of administration, and contraindications. It is the responsibility of the practitioner, relying on experience and knowledge of the patient, to determine dosages and the best treatment for each individual patient. Neither the Publisher nor the author assumes any liability for any injury and/or damage to persons or property arising from this publication.

The Publisher

ELSEVIER your source for books, journals and multimedia in the health sciences
www.elsevierhealth.com

Working together to grow
libraries in developing countries

www.elsevier.com | www.bookaid.org | www.sabre.org

ELSEVIER BOOK AID International Sabre Foundation

The publisher's policy is to use paper manufactured from sustainable forests

Printed in China
Last digit is the print number: 9 8 7 6 5 4 3 2 1

Commissioning Editor: *Sue Hodgson*
Development Editor: *Nani Clansey*
Editorial Assistant: *Rachael Harrison*
Project Manager: *Frances Affleck*
Design: *Stewart Larking*
Illustration Manager: *Gillian Richards*
Illustrator: *Jennifer Rose*
Marketing Manager(s) (UK/USA): *John Canelon/ Radha Mawrie*

Contents

Contents

Foreword

I was delighted when Mo Nahabedian asked me to write a foreword to this text on 'oncoplastic' surgery of the breast. The concept of 'oncoplastic surgery' and this textbook are evidence of an expanding sea-change in surgery and medicine. In its purest form, 'oncoplastic' surgery embodies the concept that treating the disease is no longer enough, the goal now is to treat the entire patient and to make every effort to leave the patient the same or even better than we found her. That means minimizing complications, side effects, incisions, recovery and pain. Some other examples of this same type of trend include angioplasty, laparoscopic surgery, sentinel node sampling, skin-sparing mastectomy, nipple-sparing mastectomy, and the Cyber-Knife.

Oncoplastic surgery in its original form began as combining lumpectomy or quadrantectomy with local or regional tissue rearrangement so that the breast with cancer should be conserved and reshaped so as to avoid significant deformity, particularly after radiation therapy. I would argue that the term 'oncoplastic surgery' is and should be expanded to include a philosophy that the appearance of the breast is a critical component in the treatment of breast cancer. The distinguished group of authors, including both general surgeons and plastic surgeons, who have contributed to this book all agree that women with breast cancer should be offered options to allow them to hold on to the highest quality of life possible while treating their disease.

Thus, in its broadest sense, 'oncoplastic surgery' could mean that every woman with breast cancer be offered whenever possible the following:

1. A consultation with a Plastic Surgeon
2. The option of breast conservation
3. The option of nipple-sparing or skin-sparing mastectomy
4. Oncoplastic procedures particularly for the large or pendulous breast
5. Advanced reconstructive procedures, including the latest innovations in alloplastic materials, implants and surgery, including microsurgery-assisted free-tissue transfer

The last decade has seen a number of interesting changes in the treatment of breast cancer. Two of the most interesting have been the increasing frequency of mastectomy and the increase in bilateral mastectomies. While this would seem to run counter to the narrow definition of 'oncoplastic' surgery, it fits with the broader definition of improved quality of life. As the reconstructive surgical tools have improved, the prospect of bilateral mastectomies and reconstruction has begun to look less negative than a life of endless mammograms, MRIs, suspicious X-ray findings, needle biopsies, chemotherapy, and radiation.

This text is a testament to some of the advances that have been made in breast reconstruction and 'oncoplastic' surgery. The hope is that the concepts and techniques herein described will become widely available to women and their surgeons.

Scott L Spear MD
Washington DC
2009

Preface

Oncoplastic surgery of the breast has been receiving widespread attention over the past several years. It has captured the interest of breast and plastic surgeons alike. Many women with breast cancer are excited about the possibility of removing the breast cancer, retaining important breast elements such as the nipple–areolar complex, and reconstructing a partial breast deformity all in single stage. This technique is the basis for the concept of oncoplastic breast surgery. Oncoplastic breast surgery has generated tremendous excitement over that past several years and has become an integrated component of the consultation between patients and their surgeons. As these oncoplastic techniques become more sophisticated, questions about the various applications are becoming more common. There is a clear need for surgeons and patients alike to become familiar with the indications and the available techniques in order to make oncoplastic breast surgery a safe and effective procedure. This was the impetus for preparing this important book on an evolving procedure.

Oncoplastic Surgery of the Breast represents a novel approach in the preparation of a learning tool for all surgeons interested in oncoplastic breast surgery. It has been designed to review many of the essential principles, concepts, and techniques associated with it and to provide some insight and clinical pearls that will facilitate one's ability to master these procedures. The text is structured in a 'how to' approach with a basic template that includes a large number of photographs and illustrations. The contributors for each chapter were selected based on talent, ability, reputation, and a commitment to the educational process. All of the currently available techniques for oncoplastic breast surgery are described and include reduction mammaplasty, adjacent tissue rearrangement, and the various types of flap reconstruction. The final product represents a compendium of oncoplastic operations that will be useful to all surgeons. Some of the chapters have an audiovisual component that is intended to take the reader step by step through a particular operation. It is felt that the combination of text and audiovisual material will set it apart from all previously published textbooks on oncoplastic breast surgery. It is hoped that this book will facilitate one's ability to perform these operations at a higher level of understanding and ability.

There are several individuals who were instrumental in allowing the publication of this book to come to fruition. The first are the contributing authors who prepared these outstanding chapters. These surgeons are all very busy, exceptionally talented, and have had to sacrifice a significant amount of their time for this project. I am forever indebted to them. The second are the staff at Elsevier for their hard work and commitment towards publishing this truly outstanding textbook. Finally, I would like to thank my family, Anissa, Danielle, and Sophia, for their support, patience, and understanding during the many hours spent in the preparation of this work.

Maurice Y Nahabedian MD

Contributors

Robert J Allen
Chief
Section of Plastic Surgery
Louisiana State University
Health Sciences Center
New Orleans Louisiana
USA

Elisabeth K Beahm MD FACS
Professor
Department of Reconstructive Plastic Surgery
The University of Texas MD Anderson Cancer Center
Houston, Texas
USA

Jonathan Cheng MD
Assistant Professor
Department of Plastic Surgery
University of Texas
Southwestern Medical Center
Dallas, Texas
USA

Costanza Cocilovo MD
Assistant Professor of Surgery
Department of Surgery
Georgetown University Hospital
Washington, DC
USA

Liron Eldor MD
Fellow, Plastic Surgery
Department of Plastic Surgery
The Methodist Hospital
Institute for Reconstructive Surgery
Houston, Texas
USA

Neil Fine
Associate Professor, Plastic Surgery
Division of Plastic Surgery
Northwestern University, Feinberg School of Medicine
Chicago, Illinois
USA

Moustapha Hamdi MD PhD FCCP
Professor
Department of Plastic and Reconstructive Surgery
Ghent University Hospital, Belgium
Plastic Surgeon Consultant
Edith Cavell Medical Institute
Brussels
Belgium

Catherine M Hannan MD
Resident in Plastic Surgery
Department of Surgery
Georgetown University Hospital
Washington, DC
USA

Steven J Kronowitz MD FACS
Associate Professor
Department of Plastic Surgery
The University of Texas MD Anderson Cancer Center
Houston, Texas
USA

Joshua L Levine MD
The Center for Microsurgical Breast Reconstruction
Manhattan and Charleston
New York, NY
USA

Albert Losken MD
Assistant Professor
Emory Division of Plastic and Reconstructive Surgery
Atlanta, Georgia
USA

Maurice Y Nahabedian MD FACS
Associate Professor of Plastic Surgery
Department of Plastic Surgery
Georgetown University Hospital
Washington, DC
USA

Kristina O'Shaughnessy
Chief Resident, Plastic Surgery
Division of Plastic Surgery
Northwestern University, Feinberg School of Medicine
Chicago, Illinois
USA

P Pravin Reddy MD
Private Practice
Atlanta Plastic and Reconstructive Surgery Consultants
Atlanta, Georgia
USA

Melvin J Silverstein MD FACS
Medical Director
Hoag Hospital Breast Program
Hoag Memorial Hospital Presbyterian
Newport Beach, California;
Professor of Surgery
Keck School of Medicine
University of Southern California
Los Angeles, California
USA

Anu M Singh MD
Clinical Assistant Professor
Georgetown University School of Medicine
Shady Grove Adventist Radiation Oncology Center
Rockville, Maryland
USA

Navin K Singh MD
Clinical Assistant Professor
Johns Hopkins University School of Medicine
Ivy Plastic Surgery Associates
Chevy Chase, Maryland
USA

Scott L Spear
Professor and Chairman
Department of Plastic Surgery
Georgetown University Hospital
Washington, DC
USA

Aldona J Spiegel MD
Director, Center for Breast Restoration
The Methodist Hospital
Institute for Reconstructive Surgery
Assistant Professor
Cornell University – Weill Medical School
Houston, Texas
USA

Justin West MD
Resident in Plastic Surgery
Department of Plastic Surgery
Georgetown University Hospital
Washington, DC
USA

Shawna C Willey MD FACS
Associate Professor
Director, Betty Lou Ourisman Breast Health Center
Department of Surgery
Georgetown University Hospital
Washington, DC
USA

Dedication

To my parents, Ed and Rose Nahabedian, who taught me that hard work, commitment, and perseverance are a foundation for success and happiness. To my mentors, Alan Wile, Paul Manson and Scott Spear, who have taken the time to guide and direct me on a career path that has exceeded my hopes and dreams. To these masters, I am forever grateful and indebted. To all the residents that I have had the privilege to work with at Johns Hopkins and Georgetown Universities. Their energy and enthusiasm for plastic surgery has inspired me to push the envelope and to continuously reach for the stars. To my wife Anissa, who has been my guiding light and primary support. As a result of her love, encouragement, and ability to always come up with the right answers, my life has been enriched and fulfilled. To my children, Danielle and Sophia, who have inspired me to new levels and I strive to be the father they will always love and cherish.

CHAPTER 1

History of Oncoplastic Surgery of the Breast

Maurice Y Nahabedian

Introduction

Oncoplastic surgery for the management of breast cancer has been receiving worldwide attention and gaining widespread acceptance. Simply stated, oncoplastic surgery is defined as tumor excision with a wide margin of resection followed by immediate reconstruction of the partial mastectomy defect. Much of the enthusiasm for this procedure stems from safety data demonstrating oncologic feasibility and efficacy data demonstrating high patient satisfaction. These facts, as well as others, have resulted in improved outcomes for women with breast cancer.

Although modern methods of breast cancer management date back to the turn of the 20th century, the history of oncoplastic surgery is relatively new and has not been well chronicled. There have been several paradigm shifts that have occurred over the past century regarding the various treatment modalities. (**Table 1.1**) To appreciate the current impact of oncoplastic surgery as it relates to the management of breast cancer, a brief history of modern breast cancer therapy is useful.

Prior to the era of William Stewart Halsted, the diagnosis of breast cancer was often associated with few options for management and poor patient survival. With the introduction of the radical mastectomy, the morbidity and mortality of breast cancer were markedly improved; however, the disfigurement following this operation was significant.[1] The modified radical mastectomy (MRM), in which the pectoral major muscle was preserved and the axillary lymph node basin was dissected, maintained similar survival statistics with slightly less physical disfigurement.[2-5] The simple mastectomy in conjunction with radiation therapy was introduced at the same time and continued to open the door for less aggressive surgical techniques.[6] Further refinements in mastectomy techniques allowed for skin-sparing patterns that did not modify or alter local recurrence or survival patterns.[7-9] With the introduction of sentinel lymph node biopsy for breast cancer, the need to perform an axillary dissection was significantly reduced and the simple mastectomy has become commonplace.[10,11] Finally, the application for mastectomy with preservation of the nipple–areolar complex (NAC) for malignant disease was introduced and applied for women in select situations.[12-16]

All of these mastectomy techniques resulted in significant disfigurement because the breast parenchyma was removed. In order to improve upon the physical disfigurement, breast reconstruction was introduced and popularized (**Table 1.2**). Reconstructive options have included local tissues, prosthetic devices, musculocutaneous flaps, and perforator flaps.[17-25] The evolution of these techniques has made a significant impact and ultimately led to the development of oncoplastic surgical techniques.

Table 1.1 Chronological history of operations related to total mastectomy

Author	Year	Treatment
Halsted[1]	1890	Radical mastectomy
Patey[2]	1948	Modified radical mastectomy
McWhirter[6]	1948	Simple mastectomy and radiotherapy
Toth[7]	1991	Skin-sparing mastectomy
Noguchi[10]	1996	Sentinel lymph node biopsy
VerHeyden[12]	1998	Subcutaneous mastectomy (malignant disease)

Table 1.3 Chronological history of operations related to partial mastectomy

Author	Year	Treatment
Crile[26]	1973	Partial mastectomy
Montague[28]	1978	Breast conservation therapy
Veronesi[50]	1994	Segmental parenchymal excision
Gabka[31]	1997	Oncoplastic surgery
Clough[44]	1998	Reduction mastopexy lumpectomy
Amanti[51]	2002	Periareolar parenchymal excision
Anderson[45]	2005	Parallelogram excision patterns

Table 1.2 Chronological history of operations related to breast reconstruction

Author	Year	Technique
Berson[17]	1944	Derma-fat grafts
Longacre[18]	1953	Local flaps
Snyderman[19]	1969	Prosthetic devices
Arnold[20]	1976	Omentum and prosthetics
Schneider[21]	1977	Latissimus dorsi
Hartrampf[22]	1982	TRAM flap
Argenta[23]	1984	Tissue expansion
Grotting[24]	1989	Free TRAM flap
Allen[25]	1994	Perforator flaps

TRAM, transverse rectus abdominis myocutaneous.

Over the years, as our understanding of the pathophysiology of breast cancer has improved and our utilization of radiation therapy as an adjuvant mode of therapy was optimized, modifications to these original operations have evolved (**Table 1.3**) It became accepted that for many breast cancers total mastectomy was not an absolute requirement; a partial mastectomy could be performed.[26,27] With the introduction of breast conservation therapy (BCT), breast cancers could be excised with a 2–5 mm margin, the NAC could be preserved, and breast shape and contour would be maintained in the majority of women.[28] Following the operative portion, radiation therapy is initiated. The outcomes following BCT have been generally favorable, with survival statistics that have remained essentially equal to that of MRM. However, local recurrence rates have been generally increased.[29] Although the aesthetic outcomes following BCT have been good to excellent in the majority of women, some have required secondary procedures to improve the appearance and achieve symmetry.[30] Thus, the shortcomings of BCT have included increased local recurrence and occasional breast distortion.

In an effort to reduce the incidence of local recurrence and maintain natural breast contour, the concept of oncoplastic surgery was introduced.[31,32] Oncoplastic surgery differs from standard BCT in that the margin and volume of excision are typically greater than in lumpectomy or quadrantectomy. Excision margins typically range from 1 to 2 cm and resection volumes typically range from 180 to 220 cm^3, although much greater margins and volumes are possible. The resultant deformity is reconstructed immediately using techniques related to volume replacement or volume displacement that include adjacent tissue rearrangement, reduction mammaplasty, or distant flaps. Contralateral procedures can be performed immediately at the time of partial breast reconstruction or on a delayed basis. Oncoplastic techniques have resulted in survival and local recurrence rates that are essentially equal to those of MRM.[33,34]

The purpose of this introductory chapter is to review the history of these oncoplastic procedures. This chapter will emphasize some of the landmark studies and important conclusions. It will highlight some of the surgeons who have made significant contributions to the concept and practice of oncoplastic surgery. As oncoplastic surgery continues to gain acceptance and popularity, an optimal and systematic approach to management is becoming increasingly necessary. This chapter will touch upon some of the salient components and historic vignettes of oncoplastic surgery. The subsequent chapters will expand upon many of the principles, concepts, and techniques that are important in incorporating oncoplastic surgery successfully into one's practice.

Toward safety and efficacy

The indications and patient selection criteria for oncoplastic surgery have not been without controversy, scrutiny, and criticism. There have been individuals who were of the opinion that the boundaries between oncologic management and aesthetic reconstruction have been blurred within the promotion of oncoplastic surgery.[35] Contrary to this opinion is that by adhering to oncologic principles oncoplastic techniques can be safely performed in properly selected women.[36,37] Regardless of one's opinion, in order for oncoplastic surgery to be safely and effectively performed, patients should be properly selected and properly consented for these procedures. Surgeons should be aware of all aspects relating to the recovery and well-being of these women. These include not only recurrence and survival but also donor site considerations, secondary procedures, and effects over time. The importance of proper patient counseling, with close attention to the short-term and long-term consequences, should not be dismissed. The application of these principles for ablative and reconstructive surgeons will facilitate the acceptance and success of oncoplastic surgery.

Safety in oncoplastic surgery requires attention to detail and proper technique selection. The process begins with obtaining a diagnosis. Breast cancer is diagnosed by various techniques that include fine-needle aspiration, core needle biopsy, and excisional biopsy. The next step is the excision. The importance of obtaining a clear margin becomes evident when one considers that the relative risk of developing a recurrence is 15-fold higher in patients in whom the surgical margin was not clear of tumor.[38] The question of a positive margin being related to the type of biopsy performed has been studied and found not to be related. A positive margin was, however, related to the size of the primary tumor (T3 > T2 > T1) and to histological subtype (lobular > ductal).[37] Preoperative identification of those women with infiltrating lobular carcinoma who may be at higher risk of a positive surgical margin can be sometimes made via mammography based on the presence of architectural distortion.[39]

In light of the fact that larger tumors have an increased likelihood of a positive margin, the benefit of oncoplastic resections has been recognized. It has been demonstrated by Kaur, et al that resection margins are greater and the incidence of a positive margin is reduced when comparing oncoplastic resection to standard quadrantectomy.[40] Mean resection volume in this study was 200 cm^3 following oncoplastic resection and 117 cm^3 following quadrantectomy. Giacalone, et al have demonstrated that glandular resection was increased, histological margins

were wider, and the need for re-excision was decreased following oncoplastic surgery.[41] There was a trend toward fewer mastectomies following oncoplastic resection (2/42, 4.8%) compared to standard lumpectomy (12/57, 21.1%). These facts are merely scratching the surface regarding the safety and efficacy of oncoplastic surgery. Additional studies and supportive data will be reviewed in the upcoming chapters.

Immediate reconstruction of the partial mastectomy deformity

The techniques that are currently used for the reconstruction of the partial mastectomy defect are based on two different concepts: volume displacement and volume replacement. Volume displacement procedures include local tissue rearrangement, reduction mammaplasty, and mastopexy. Volume replacement procedures include local and remote flaps from various regions of the body. All of these techniques have been utilized extensively and found to be useful. The indications for each are different and various algorithms have been devised to assist with the decision process.[42–44] In these studies, the selection of appropriate technique was based primarily on bra cup size and defect size. In general, women with smaller breasts with minimal ptosis were found to be better candidates for volume replacement procedures, e.g. local flap, latissimus dorsi, lateral thoracic flap; whereas women with larger and more ptotic breasts would be better candidates for volume displacement procedures, e.g. adjacent tissue rearrangement, reduction mammaplasty, mastopexy. The history of these techniques as they relate to oncoplastic surgery will be further reviewed (Table 1.4).

Reduction mammaplasty

It is difficult to state with certainty who first began performing immediate partial breast reconstruction; however, the individual who is most credited with the introduction and popularization is Melvin J Silverstein MD. This

Table 1.4 Synopsis of oncoplastic procedures and their relation to morbidity and patient satisfaction

Study	Year	Technique	#	Morbidity	Satisfaction
Kat[53]	1999	Latissimus dorsi	30	38% (seroma, infection)	100%
Losken[49]	2002	Reduction mammaplasty	20	30% (delayed healing)	100%
Clough[46]	2003	Reduction mammaplasty	101	20% (delayed healing, fibrosis)	88%
Gendy[55]	2003	Latissimus dorsi	47	8% (sensory changes, reduction in ADL)	84%
Spear[48]	2003	Reduction mammaplasty	11	27% (fat necrosis)	100%
Losken[54]	2004	Latissimus dorsi	30	33% (recurrence, seroma)	NA

ADL, activities of daily living; NA, not applicable.

occurred in 1982 following the excision of a fibro-adenoma. The breast was immediately repaired using a reduction mammaplasty approach.[45]

Since then, reduction mammaplasty has been frequently utilized for oncoplastic surgery.[44–47] There have been several studies that have reported on outcomes (**Table 1.5**). Krishna Clough MD has been a significant contributor and proponent of oncoplastic resection. He began performing reduction-based oncoplastic operations in the 1980s and recently reported on his 14-year experience from the Curie Institute in Paris, France.[42,44,46] Subjects included 101 women who were selected for oncoplastic resection because a standard lumpectomy would have resulted in a significant contour abnormality. The primary reduction technique utilized was an inverted 'T' with the NAC based on a superior pedicle. The contralateral reduction mammaplasty was performed immediately in 83% of women and secondarily in 17% of women. Mean tumor excision weight was 222 g. The 5-year local recurrence rate was 9.4%, the overall survival rate was 95.7%, and the metastasis-free survival rate was 82.8%. Cosmetic outcome was satisfactory in 82% of women. It was demonstrated that cosmetic outcome tended to deteriorate when radiotherapy was delivered preoperatively compared to postoperatively.

Scott Spear MD, et al have reported on their 6-year experience from 1996 to 2002, combining wide excision of tumor with immediate bilateral reduction mammaplasty.[48] These operations were all performed in a multidisciplinary fashion. All women in this cohort had large breasts and wore 'D' cup brassières. The mean excision volume was 1085 g per breast. Follow-up ranged from 1 to 6 years with a mean of 24 months. No woman developed a local recurrence, although one woman died of metastatic disease. Complications included fat necrosis ($n = 3$), nipple hypopigmentation ($n = 2$), hematoma, and complex scar. Patient satisfaction was scored on a visual analog scale that ranged from 1 to 4 with a mean score of 3.3. A panel of independent observers also graded the outcomes and scored the pre-radiation outcome as 2.9 and the post-radiation outcome as 3.03. The principal conclusions from this study were that oncoplastic resection of tumor followed by immediate bilateral reduction mammaplasty avoided the significant asymmetry that would occur following BCT alone or following total mastectomy with immediate total breast reconstruction. Another important conclusion was that the combination of wide excision with immediate reconstruction was oncologically safe.

Albert Losken MD and the group at Emory University in Atlanta, Georgia, have reported on their 10-year (1991–2000) experience utilizing reduction mammaplasty in the setting of oncoplastic surgery.[43,49] A total of 20 women were included in this review. Mean tumor size was 1.5 mm and the mean weight of the tumor specimen was 288 g. The excised surgical margins were negative in 80%. The most common reduction technique was a superomedial or inferior pedicle. Postoperative abnormal mammograms were noted in 8 women (40%), all of whom underwent additional biopsy. No woman was noted to have a recurrence with a mean follow-up of 23 months. Breast aesthetics and patient satisfaction was acceptable in all women.

These studies, as well as others, have demonstrated the utility of reduction mammaplasty in the setting of oncoplastic surgery. Because the techniques are variable and a greater attention to operative detail is necessary with reduction mammaplasty, a two-team approach is advocated. The contralateral breast is usually reduced simultaneously; however, when obtaining a clear surgical margin is uncertain, a delayed approach can be safely performed.

Adjacent tissue rearrangement

Adjacent tissue rearrangement is perhaps the most common method by which the partial mastectomy defect is reconstructed. This is because these techniques rarely require a two-team approach as the ablative surgeon will apply the principles and techniques to close these defects. The specific techniques fall within the domain of volume displacement procedures. These techniques are primarily indicated when the partial deformity extends to the chest

Table 1.5 Synopsis of oncoplastic reduction mammaplasty and its relation to oncologic and aesthetic outcomes

Study	Year	Technique	Patients	Tumor size (cm)	Follow-up (months)	Margin involvement (%)	Local recurrence (%)	Cosmetic failure (%)
Chang[68]	2004	Reduction mammaplasty	37	0.6–5.2	NR	2.7	0	NR
Spear[48]	2003	Reduction mammaplasty	11	NR	24	0	0	NR
Clough[46]	2003	Reduction mammaplasty	101	3.2	46	10.9	6.9	12
Newman[70]	2001	Reduction mammaplasty	28	1.5	24	7	0	NR
Nos[71]	1998	Reduction mammaplasty	50	3.25	48	10	7	15

NR, not recorded.

wall and there is sufficient adjacent tissue to close the defect and maintain a natural contour. Volume replacement techniques are usually not necessary because there is sufficient local tissue. Although several surgeons have described various volume displacement techniques, it is generally accepted that Melvin Silverstein MD was one of the pioneers who introduced and popularized the concepts.[45]

The need to develop these volume displacement techniques stems from the fact that traditional methods of lumpectomy and closure frequently resulted in a contour abnormality of the breast. The reason was that the excision was confined to the lesion and not the surrounding parenchyma. Adjacent tissues were not adequately mobilized and the excision defect was closed primarily. With these volume displacement techniques, the excision is usually extended to the chest wall and the adjacent parenchyma is undermined and mobilized in order to permit the closure of small or large deformities without creating a contour abnormality. **Table 1.6** reviews several of the volume displacement techniques.

There are several pioneers who deserve credit and mention in the evolution of these techniques. Veronesi and colleagues introduced the concept of segmental parenchymal wide excision including the overlying skin.[50] This allowed for the quadrantectomy approach, which was instrumental in establishing the feasibility of breast conservation therapy. These operations were generally performed using a radial approach for tumors that were laterally based. An alternative to the radial approach was the periareolar approach initially described by Amanti, et al.[51] This permitted excisions that resulted in less conspicuous scars. With the introduction of periareolar subcutaneous quadrantectomy, also known as periareolar donut mastopexy, incisions could be created circumferentially around the NAC and remain relatively inconspicuous. Silverstein has introduced various concepts that include skin incisions using a parallelogram pattern and batwing mastopexy.[45] These parallelogram incisions allowed for wider excision margins while maintaining the natural contour of the breast. Batwing mastopexy is an extension of this concept and is used primarily for centrally situated tumors near the NAC. Clough, et al have

Table 1.6 Options for oncoplastic adjacent tissue rearrangement based on tumor location and distribution. Reproduced with permission from Anderson BO, Masetti R, Silverstein ML. Oncoplastic approaches to the partial mastectomy: an overview of volume displacement techniques. Lancet Oncol 2005; 6:145–157

Type of lumpectomy	Tumor location	Tumor distribution
Batwing mastopexy	Central breast	Localized
Radial segment quadrantectomy	Lateral breast	Extended
Donut mastopexy	Upper or lateral breast	Extended
Reduction mastopexy	Lower breast	Localized

introduced the technique of reduction mastopexy lumpectomy.[46] This technique has been especially useful for tumors situated near the lower pole of the breast. Standard lumpectomy of these tumors would often result in an inferiorly displaced NAC. All of these techniques have specific indications based on tumor location that are highlighted in Table 1.6.

Local and remote flaps

Local and remote flaps fall within the domain of volume replacement procedures. These options have been most useful for defects in which volume displacement procedures would not be adequate owing to breast volume considerations or extent of resection. There are several options that have been useful. The selection of one technique versus another will depend upon the abilities of the reconstructive surgeon and include musculocutaneous flaps and perforator flaps that can be transferred on a vascularized pedicle or as a free tissue transfer. Many of these options will be reviewed in subsequent chapters. What is provided in this chapter is a brief overview of the techniques and their origins.

The most commonly used flap for immediate reconstruction of the partial mastectomy defect has been the latissimus dorsi musculocutaneous flap.[52-57] This flap has been effectively used for deformities of the superior, lateral and inferior aspects of the breasts (**Table 1.7**). In

Table 1.7 Synopsis of oncoplastic latissimus dorsi flap reconstruction and its relationship to oncologic and aesthetic outcomes

Study	Year	Technique	Patients	Tumor size (cm)	Follow-up (months)	Margin involvement (%)	Local recurrence (%)	Cosmetic failure (%)
Dixon[67]	2002	Latissimus dorsi	25	NR	NR	0	NR	NR
Kat[53]	1999	Latissimus dorsi	30	NR	NR	0	NR	NR
Gendy[55]	2003	Latissimus dorsi	49	2.2	53	0	4	1.8
Nano[69]	2004	Latissimus dorsi	18	3	24	5.5	0	5.5
Losken[54]	2004	Latissimus dorsi	39	NR	44	0	5.1	NR

NR: not recorded.

general, a two-team approach is needed for this operation owing to the technical aspects in designing, elevating, and mobilizing the flap. There have been several methods described by which the latissimus dorsi flap can be harvested. The traditional technique incorporated a posterolateral thoracic incision, whereas the more modern technique utilizes an endoscope.[54,57] With the endoscopic technique the muscle is accessed through the breast and axillary incision. No skin is removed. Kat, et al have reviewed their 3-year experience from 1994 to 1996 in 30 women who had oncoplastic surgery using the latissimus dorsi musculocutaneous flap.[53] All women had tumors located in the superior, lateral, or inferior quadrants. There were no centrally located tumors. All patients demonstrated total flap survival and were all pleased with the aesthetic outcome. Losken, et al have reviewed their 5-year experience from 1994 to 1998 using the latissimus dorsi muscle flap harvested endoscopically in 39 women.[54] Donor site morbidities occurred in 12 women (31%) and included a seroma in 7 women as well as skin necrosis, lymphedema, dehiscence, hypertrophic scarring, and a persistent sinus tract.

Another method of harvesting the latissimus dorsi is as a mini-flap.[55,56] The advantage of the mini-flap is that variable amounts of the latissimus dorsi muscle can be harvested based on the volume requirements of the breast. The flap is generally harvested through an extended anterolateral breast incision that is used for the resection as well. Rainsbury has used this flap extensively and feels that it is highly useful because it extends the role of BCT and oncoplastic surgery, enables reconstruction for a deformity involving 20–30% of the breast, can be used for central, upper inner and upper outer quadrant tumors, and finally can be performed immediately or on a delayed basis.[56] Gendy, et al have used the latissimus dorsi mini-flap in 89 women between 1991 and 1999.[55] Outcomes were compared to skin-sparing mastectomy and immediate reconstruction. Findings were favorable for the oncoplastic techniques with regard to postoperative complications (8% vs 14%), further surgical interventions (12% vs 79%), nipple sensory loss (2% vs 98%), restricted activities (54% vs 73%), and cosmetic outcome (visual analog score: 83.5 vs 72).

The use of perforator flaps for the reconstruction of the partial mastectomy has been receiving increasing attention. There are three flaps that have been used for this purpose: the thoracodorsal artery perforator flap (TDAP), the lateral thoracic flap, and the intercostal perforator flap.[58–62] The TDAP is an adipocutaneous flap in which the latissimus dorsi muscle is totally spared. The vascularity of the flap is derived from the perforating branches of the thoracodorsal artery and vein. The lateral thoracic flap is a fasciocutaneous flap that is perfused via either the lateral thoracic, axillary, or thoracodorsal artery and vein. The intercostal perforator flap is usually perfused via a perforating intercostal artery and vein that is based along the inferior aspect of the anterior axillary line. These flaps are usually transferred on a vascularized pedicle but may be transferred as a free tissue transfer as well.

Clinical experience with these flaps has been encouraging. Levine, et al have provided an algorithm for perforator flap utilization.[58] The first choice is the TDAP flap, followed by the lateral thoracic flap, and finally the intercostal perforator flap. The decision is based on the quality of the vessels during the operative procedure. Munhoz, et al have used the lateral thoracic flap in 34 women for partial breast reconstruction.[61] Flap complications included partial necrosis in three (8.8%), which included fat necrosis that developed in 2 women. Another woman developed an infection. Donor site complications included a seroma in 5 women (14.7%) and wound dehiscence in 3 women (8.8%). Patient satisfaction was achieved in 88% of women with a mean follow-up period of 23 months.

Breast reconstruction following mastectomy with nipple–areolar preservation

Nipple–areolar preservation in the setting of mastectomy is perhaps the most recent oncoplastic technique. Although this operation includes a total mastectomy rather than partial mastectomy, it is considered by many to be an oncoplastic procedure because the NAC is preserved. This has been the topic of some controversy because the general indications for mastectomy are that the tumor characteristics are such that a partial mastectomy is deemed relatively unsafe due to tumor size, location, or lymph node status. In these cases, the fear is that the NAC may be a harbinger of tumor cells. Previous studies have demonstrated that the incidence of tumor involvement of the NAC ranges from 12% to 58%.[63,64] Lambert, et al have reviewed the factors that are predictive of nipple involvement in a study of 803 women.[65] The factors that were statistically significant predictors of tumor involvement included advanced stage (III, IV), tumor size (>5 cm), number of positive lymph nodes, central or overlapping locations, and undifferentiated tumors. Laronga, et al at the MD Anderson cancer center have evaluated NAC involvement in 326 women having skin-sparing mastectomy and found an incidence of occult involvement in 5.6%.[66] They found no difference in positivity based on tumor size, nuclear grade, or histological subtype.

The clinical experience following breast reconstruction in the setting of nipple–areolar preservation has been somewhat mixed but with a favorable trend.[13,14,16] Clearly, patient selection has been a critical determinant of outcome based on aesthetic and oncologic considerations. Nahabedian and Tsangaris have evaluated the aesthetic outcomes following NAC preservation in 14 breasts and demonstrated that areolar sensation was present in 43%, delayed healing of the NAC in 28%, NAC asymmetry in 50%, and secondary procedures related to the

NAC in 36%.[13] In 11/14 breasts, the reconstruction was in the setting of breast cancer with a local recurrence in 3/11 (27%). Despite these morbidities, patient satisfaction was achieved in 78% of women. Sacchini, et al have demonstrated a very low recurrence with an occurrence in 2/64 (3.1%).[16] No woman had tumor involvement of the NAC. Satisfaction scores were good to excellent in 87% of women who had cancer and 94% in women who did not have breast cancer.

Conclusion

This introductory chapter has been intended to review the history of oncoplastic surgery and to provide a framework for the remaining chapters. All of the principles, concepts, and specific techniques will be discussed in greater detail in the forthcoming chapters.

References

1. Halsted WS. The results of radical operations for the cure of breast carcinoma. Ann Surg 1894; 20:497.

2. Patey DH. The treatment of malignant disease: surgery. Middx Hosp J 1948; 48:111–115.

3. Madden JL. Modified radical mastectomy. Surg Gynecol Obstet 1965; 121:1221–1230.

4. Donegan WL, Sugarbaker ED, Handley RS, et al. The management of primary operable breast cancer: a comparison of time–mortality factors after standard, extended, and modified radical mastectomy. Proc Natl Cancer Conf. 1970; 6:135–143.

5. Scanlon EF, Caprini JA. Modified radical mastectomy. Cancer 1975; 35:710–713.

6. McWhirter R. The value of simple mastectomy and radiotherapy in the treatment of cancer of the breast. Br J Radiol 1948; 21:599–610.

7. Toth BA, Lappert P. Modified skin incisions for mastectomy: the need for plastic surgical input in preoperative planning. Plast Reconstr Surg 1991; 87:1048–1053.

8. Singletary SE. Skin-sparing mastectomy with immediate breast reconstruction: the MD Anderson Cancer Center experience. Ann Surg Oncol 1996; 3:411–416.

9. Slavin S, Schnitt SJ, Duda R, et al. Skin-sparing mastectomy and immediate reconstruction: oncologic risks and aesthetic results in patients with early-stage breast cancer. Plast Reconstr Surg 1998; 102:49–62.

10. Noguchi M, Katev N, Myazaki I. Diagnosis of axillary lymph node metastases in patients with breast cancer. Breast Cancer Res Treat 1996; 40:283–293.

11. O'Hea BJ, Hill AD, El Shirbini AM, et al. Sentinel lymph node biopsy in breast cancer: initial experience at Memorial Sloan-Kettering Cancer Center. J Am Coll Surg 1998; 186:423–427.

12. VerHeyden CN. Nipple-sparing total mastectomy of large breasts: the role of tissue expansion. Plast Reconstr Surg 1998; 101:1494–1500.

13. Nahabedian MY, Tsangaris TN. Breast reconstruction following subcutaneous mastectomy for cancer: a critical appraisal of the nipple–areolar complex. Plast Reconstr Surg 2006; 117:1083–1090.

14. Crowe JP, Kim JA, Yetman R, et al. Nipple-sparing mastectomy technique and results of 54 procedures. Arch Surg 2004; 139:148–150.

15. Cense HA, Rutgers EJ, Lopes Cardozo M, et al. Nipple-sparing mastectomy in breast cancer: a viable option? EJSO 2001; 27:521–526.

16. Sacchini V, Pinotti JA, Barros A, et al. Nipple-sparing mastectomy for breast cancer and risk reduction: oncologic or technical problem? J Am Coll Surg 2006; 203:704–714.

17. Berson MI. Derma-fat-fascia transplants used in building up the breasts. Surgery 1944; 15:451.

18. Longacre JJ. The use of local pedicle flaps for reconstruction of the breast after total or subtotal extirpation of the mammary gland and for correction of distortion and atrophy of the breast due to excessive scar. Plast Reconstr Surg 1953; 11:380.

19. Snyderman RK, Guthrie RH. Reconstruction of the female breast following radical mastectomy. Plast Reconstr Surg 1971; 47:465.

20. Arnold PG, Hartrampf CA, Jurkiewicz MJ. One-stage reconstruction of the breast, using the transposed greater omentum. Case report. Plast Reconstr Surg 1976; 57:520–522.

21. Schneider WJ, Hill HL Jr, Brown RG. Latissimus dorsi myocutaneous flap for breast reconstruction. Br J Plast Surg 1977; 30:277.

22. Hartrampf CR, Scheflan M, Black PW. Breast reconstruction with a transverse abdominal island flap. Plast Reconstr Surg 1982; 69:216–225.

23. Argenta LC. Reconstruction of the breast by tissue expansion. Clin Plast Surg 1984; 11:257–264.

24. Grotting JC, Urist MM, Maddox WA, et al. Conventional TRAM flap versus free microsurgical TRAM flap for immediate breast reconstruction. Plast Reconstr Surg 1989; 83:828–841.

25. Allen RJ, Treece P. Deep inferior epigastric perforator flap for breast reconstruction. Ann Plast Surg 1994; 32:32–38.

26. Crile G, Esselstyn CB, Hermann RE, et al. Partial mastectomy for carcinoma of the breast. Surg Gynecol Obstet 1973; 136:929–933.

27. Crile G. Results of conservative treatment of breast cancer at ten and 15 years. Ann Surg 1975; 181:26–30.

28. Montague E, Gutierrez AE, Barker JL, et al. Conservation surgery and irradiation for the treatment of favorable breast cancer. Cancer 1979; 43:1058–1061.

29. Fisher B, Anderson S, Bryant J, et al. Twenty-year follow-up of a randomized trial comparing total mastectomy, lumpectomy, and lumpectomy plus irradiation for the treatment of invasive breast cancer. N Engl J Med 2002; 347:1233–1241.

30. Matory WE, Wertheimer M, Fitzgerald TJ. Aesthetic results following partial mastectomy and radiation therapy. Plast Reconstr Surg 1990; 85:739–746.

31. Gabka CJ, Maiwald G, Baumeister RG. Expanding the indications spectrum for breast saving therapy of breast carcinoma by oncoplastic operations. Langenbecks Arch Chir Suppl Kongressbd 1997; 114:1224–1227.

32. Masetti R, Pirulli PG, Magno S, et al. Oncoplastic techniques in the conservative surgical treatment of breast cancer. Breast Cancer 2000; 7:276–280.

33. Rietjens M, Urban CA, Rey PC, et al. Long-term oncological results of breast conservative treatment with oncoplastic surgery. Breast 2007; 16:387–395.

34. Asgeirsson KS, Rasheed T, McCulley SJ, et al. Oncological and cosmetic outcomes of oncoplastic breast conserving surgery. Eur J Surg Oncol 2005; 31:817–823.

35. Rew DA. Towards a scientific basic for oncoplastic breast surgery (editorial). EJSO 2003; 29:105–106.

36. Benson JR, Querci Della Rovere G. Towards a scientific basis for oncoplastic breast surgery (reply). Eur J Surg Oncol 2003; 29:629.

37. Chapgar AB, Martin RCG, Hagendoorn LJ, et al. Lumpectomy margins are affected by tumor size and histologic subtype but not by biopsy technique. Am J Surg 2004; 188:399–402.

38. Schnitt SJ, Abner A, Gelman R, et al. The relationship between microscopic margins of resection and the risk of local recurrence in patients treated with

breast conserving surgery and radiation therapy. Cancer 1994; 74:1746–1751.

39. Moore MM, Borossa G, Imbrie JZ, et al. Association of infiltrating lobular carcinoma with positive surgical margins after breast-conservation therapy. Ann Surg 2000; 231:877–882.

40. Kaur N, Petit JY, Rietjens M, et al. Comparative study of surgical margins in oncoplastic surgery and quadrantectomy in breast cancer. Ann Surg Oncol 2005; 12:1–7.

41. Giacalone PL, Roger P, Dubon O, et al. Lumpectomy vs oncoplastic surgery for breast-conserving therapy of cancer: a prospective study about 99 patients. Ann Chir 2006; 131:256–261.

42. Kronowitz SJ, Feledy JA, Hunt KK. Determining the optimal approach to breast reconstruction after partial mastectomy. Plast Reconstr Surg 2006; 117:1–11.

43. Losken A, Styblo TM, Carlson GW, et al. Management algorithm and outcome evaluation of partial mastectomy defects treated using reduction or mastopexy techniques. Ann Plast Surg 2007; 59:235–242.

44. Clough KB, Cuminet J, Fitoussi A, et al. Cosmetic sequelae after conservative treatment for breast cancer: classification and results of surgical correction. Ann Plast Surg 1998; 41:471–481.

45. Anderson BO, Masetti R, Silverstein ML. Oncoplastic approaches to the partial mastectomy: an overview of volume displacement techniques. Lancet Oncol 2005; 6:145–157.

46. Clough KB, Lewis JS, Couturaud B, et al. Oncoplastic techniques allow extensive resections for breast-conserving therapy of breast carcinomas. Ann Surg 2003; 237:26–34.

47. Munhoz AM, Montag E, Arruda EG, et al. Critical analysis of reduction mammaplasty techniques in combination with breast conservation surgery for early breast cancer treatment. Plast Reconstr Surg 2006; 117:1091–1103.

48. Spear SL, Pelletiere CV, Wolfe AJ, et al. Experience with reduction mammaplasty combined with breast conservation therapy in the management of breast cancer. Plast Reconstr Surg 2003; 111:1102–1109.

49. Losken A, Elwood ET, Styblo TM, et al. The role of reduction mammaplasty in correcting partial mastectomy defects. Plast Reconstr Surg 2002; 109:968–975.

50. Veronesi U, Luini A, Galimberti V, et al. Conservation approaches for the management of stage I/II carcinoma of the breast: Milan Cancer Institute trials. World J Surg 1994; 18:70–75.

51. Amanti C, Moscaroli A, Lo Russo M, et al. Periareolar subcutaneous quadrantectomy: a new approach in breast cancer surgery. G Chir 2002; 23:445–449.

52. Noguchi M, Taniya T, Miyazaki I, et al. Immediate transposition of a latissimus dorsi muscle for correcting a postquadrantectomy breast deformity in Japanese patients. Int Surg 1990; 75:166–170.

53. Kat CC, Darcy CM, O'Donoghue JM, et al. The use of the latissimus dorsi flap for the immediate correction of the deformity resulting from breast conserving therapy. Br J Plast Surg 1999; 52:99–103.

54. Losken A, Schaefer TG, Carlson GW, et al. Immediate endoscopic latissimus dorsi flap. Ann Plast Surg 2004; 53:1–5.

55. Gendy RK, Able JA, Rainsbury RM. Impact of skin sparing mastectomy with immediate reconstruction and breast sparing reconstruction with miniflaps on the outcomes of oncoplastic breast surgery. Br J Surg 2003; 90:433–439.

56. Rainsbury RM. Breast sparing reconstruction with latissimus dorsi miniflaps. EJSO 2002; 28:891–895.

57. Monticciolo DL, Ross D, Bostwick J 3rd, et al. Autologous breast reconstruction with endoscopic latissimus dorsi musculosubcutaneous flaps in patients choosing breast-conserving therapy: mammographic appearance. Am J Roentgenol 1996; 167:385–389.

58. Levine JL, Soueid NE, Allen RJ. Algorithm for autologous breast reconstruction for partial mastectomy defects. Plast Reconstr Surg 2005; 116:762–767.

59. Holmstrom H, Lossing C. The lateral thoracodorsal flap in breast reconstruction. Plast Reconstr Surg 1986; 577:933.

60. Holmstrom H, Lossing C. Lateral thoracodorsal flap: an intercostal perforator flap for breast reconstruction. Semin Plast Surg 2002; 16:53.

61. Munhoz A, Montag E, Arruda EG, et al. The role of the lateral thoracodorsal fasciocutaneous flap in immediate conservative breast surgery reconstruction. Plast Reconstr Surg 2006; 116:1699–1710.

62. Angrigiani C, Grilli D, Siebert J. Latissimus dorsi musculocutaneous flap without muscle. Plast Reconstr Surg 1995; 96:1608–1614.

63. Santini D, Taffurelli M, Carolina G, et al. Neoplastic involvement of nipple–areolar complex in invasive breast cancer. Am J Surg 1989; 158:399–402.

64. Menon RS, van Geel AN. Cancer of the breast with nipple involvement. Br J Cancer 1989; 59:81–84.

65. Lambert PA, Kolm P, Perry RR. Parameters that predict nipple involvement in breast cancer. J Am Coll Surg 2000; 191:354–359.

66. Laronga C, Kemp B, Johnston D, et al. Incidence of occult nipple–areola complex involvement in breast cancer patients receiving a skin-sparing mastectomy. Ann Surg Oncol 1999; 6:609–613.

67. Dixon JM, Venizelos B, Chan P. Latissimus dorsi miniflap: a new technique for extending breast conservation. Breast 2002; 11:58–65.

68. Chang E, Johnson N, Webber B, et al. Bilateral reduction mammaplasty in combination with lumpectomy for treatment of breast cancer in patients with macromastia. Am J Surg 2004; 187:647–651.

69. Nano TM, Grantley Gill P, Kollias J, et al. Breast volume replacement using the latissimus dorsi miniflap. ANZ J Surg 2004; 74:98–104.

70. Newman LA, Kuerer HM, McNeese MD, et al. Reduction mammoplasty improves breast conservation therapy in patients with macromastia. Am J Surg 2001; 181:215–220.

71. Nos C, Fitoussi A, Bourgeois D, et al. Conservative treatment of lower pole breast cancers by bilateral mammoplasty and radiotherapy. Eur J Surg Oncol 1998; 24:508–514.

CHAPTER 2

Oncoplastic Surgery: Safety and Efficacy

Costanza Cocilovo • Shawna C Willey

Introduction

For most of the 20th century, mastectomy was the surgical treatment of choice for breast cancer. Mastectomy is a disfiguring operation. Umberto Veronesi introduced breast conservation in the 1970s and has shown with multiple long-term studies that breast-conserving surgery has overall similar survival to mastectomy with a higher local recurrence rate. The rationale for considering breast-conserving surgery followed by radiation therapy came from several studies conducted in the 1970s and 1980s. From 1973 to 1980, the Milan Cancer Institute recruited patients for a randomized study to compare radical mastectomy with breast-conserving surgery termed 'quadrantectomy'. Quadrantectomy, as the name implies, involves removing a quarter of the breast. There were 701 patients enrolled in the study who had invasive breast cancers with a maximum diameter of 2 cm or less and no palpable axillary nodes. Of these, 352 were randomized to breast conservation. All patients had a complete axillary dissection and radiation if they underwent breast conservation. Results at 20 years showed overall and breast cancer specific survival rates were similar in the two groups. Local recurrences were higher in the group that received breast-conserving therapy.[1] The Milan Trial II was designed to compare 'tumorectomy' with axillary dissection and radiation therapy to 'quadrantectomy' with axillary dissection and radiation. A tumorectomy in this study is defined as excision of the tumor with a 2 mm margin of healthy tissue around it. The overall survival rate was not different in the two groups but the local recurrence rate in the tumorectomy group (13.3%) was twice that of the quadrantectomy (5.3%) group. Local recurrence was highest in patients with an extensive intraductal component.[2]

The challenge is how to select which patients are best served by breast conservation and how to achieve balance between the need for a proper oncologic operation with an acceptable cosmetic result. In Europe, quadrantectomy is often favored because of its lower local recurrence rate; however, a larger volume of breast tissue is removed. The goal is to find a way to preserve the symmetry, shape and contour of the breast, while allowing these more aggressive resections to widely clear margins. Oncoplastic surgery attempts to do this. Oncoplastic surgery is the concept of combining a plastic surgery procedure with breast-conserving surgery to achieve a more favorable final cosmetic result without compromising oncologic principles. It is a broad term that covers tissue rearrangement within the patient's breast, the use of prosthetic devices to supplement tissue, or the creation of additional volume by adding a native tissue flap. Many questions then arise: Who needs these reconstructive techniques? Should they be performed with muscle flaps or tissue rearrangement? When should they be performed? Should they be performed at the time of the original surgery; in an immediate–delayed fashion

2–3 weeks after the original surgery, or after radiation therapy is complete? What happens to patients who have positive margins after their original surgery? The following sections will review these reconstructive options.

Muscle flap

Losken et al reported on their series of 39 patients who underwent lumpectomy or quadrantectomy with immediate latissimus reconstruction. The average follow-up was 3.7 years. Four patients with DCIS (ductal carcinoma in situ) and 5 with invasive carcinoma had positive or inadequate margins. Two DCIS patients underwent re-excision and confirmation of negative margins. Of the 5 patients with invasive cancer, 2 had re-excision to clear margins, and 1 had a re-excision to negative margins but had a local recurrence 2 years later and underwent a mastectomy (**Table 2.1**).

The authors reported no interference in follow-up imaging or physical examination in the diagnosis of local recurrence due to the flap. Several patients required resection of the latissimus flap to achieve local control of the tumor because of positive margins or tumor recurrence, causing loss of a useful muscle flap and significant morbidity. Not including patients with known metastatic disease at the time of original surgery, 7 of 39 patients (18%) lost their flap. The authors concluded that it was oncologically safer to not perform immediate latissimus transposition into a fresh lumpectomy site given this rate of flap losses.[3] The need to have clear margins when performing breast conservation is important; however, with immediate oncoplastic surgery the need is imperative. An immediate flap reconstruction is not advised without having clearly established negative margins.

Tissue rearrangement

One of the largest series of tissue rearrangement procedures was reported by Clough et al, at the Institut Curie between July 1985 and June 1999. There were 101 consecutive women with breast carcinoma who underwent wide lumpectomy with tissue remodeling and mammaplasty as well as a contralateral symmetry procedure. Patients with large tumors in whom a standard lumpec-

tomy would have been deforming but in whom clear margins could be obtained with a larger resection were chosen. Eighty-nine women had an immediate contralateral procedure and 12 women had a delayed procedure. On the affected side, 11 patients had involved margins. Six patients had a mastectomy and 5 had a boost to the tumor bed with no re-excision of margins. 20% of patients had an early complication. These complications included hematoma, seroma, abscess, delayed wound healing, skin necrosis, and nipple–areolar necrosis. Four patients required reoperation and 4 patients with delayed wound healing had a delay in radiation treatment. Seven patients developed a local recurrence, 4 of which were in the same quadrant, for a rate of 9.4% (**Fig. 2.1**).

At a median follow-up of 46 months, 13 patients developed distant metastases. 88% of patients had acceptable cosmetic results (rated as excellent, good, or fair). In patients with poor results the most frequently cited flaw is that the residual breast volume is too small. Results were worse in patients who had received preoperative chemotherapy, as these patients had larger volumes resected. The authors concluded that their results demonstrate the feasibility of performing large resections and using local tissue rearrangement to fill the deficit. Their survival rates are comparable to large trials. The median weight of tissue removed was 222 g. With this amount, it was feasible to follow standard treatment protocols and to reconstruct the breast in an acceptable fashion.[4]

Role of surgical margins

These authors, as in most series, report a local recurrence rate and a rate of metastases but do not clarify how much overlap there is between these groups. We know that inadequate margins lead to higher local recurrence rates. Recurrence rates as high as 17% have been reported when local excision was incomplete.[5] We do know if inadequate resections lead to a higher rate of distant metastases or if those 5 patients with inadequate margins, who received a boost rather than a mastectomy, had their cancer care compromised by the decision. The authors were aiming

Positive margins at time of original surgery	Lost latissimus flap
9	3 (7.6%)

Developed local or distant recurrence	Lost latissimus flap
6	4 (10.2%)

Table 2.1

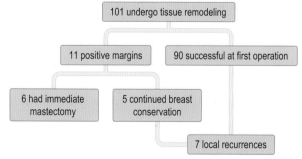

Figure 2.1

for 1 cm margins and report that many of their patients had a wider rim. These wider excisions are beneficial from the oncologic point of view as they decrease the risk of local recurrence. They are also important when patients undergo neoadjuvant chemotherapy, because even when there is a response the tumor may shrink in a multi-focal fashion and a large resection still needs to be performed.[4]

Cosmesis and follow-up

Clough et al reported that clinical and radiologic follow-up was not affected in this group. Large-breasted women often have more post-radiation changes. Several reasons are offered for this: greater dose inhomogeneity, poorer daily set-up reproduction, and increased fat content resulting in greater fibrosis. By decreasing breast size and reducing the overall volume requiring radiation, onco-plastic surgery could have a positive effect.

The authors also cite a reduction in the breast cancer risk by performing contralateral reduction. Although there are some retrospective studies that support this claim,[6] we do not currently recommend breast reduction as a form of risk reduction for breast cancer. The use of magnetic resonance imaging (MRI) in patients with a new diagnosis has been shown to detect approximately 3% of otherwise undetected contralateral primary cancers.[7] As the use of MRI increases, undetected contralateral primaries will be less of an issue.

Increased operative time is certainly a factor in performing oncoplastic surgery, and the longer duration and greater extent of surgery lead to more complications. The number of patients whose chemotherapy or radiation was delayed was approximately 4%.[4] The usual recommendation is to start the next treatment within 6 weeks of the original surgery, although data vary on what is an optimal length of time. A staged approach, especially for the contralateral breast, could decrease the possibility of a delay of adjuvant therapy. If a patient requires chemotherapy, the oncoplastic portion can be performed after chemotherapy but before radiation therapy. In patients who will not receive chemotherapy, waiting 2 or 3 weeks and then performing the reconstructive portion once margins have been cleared is an option.

Immediate versus delayed reconstruction

Kronowitz et al have reported on their experience with 69 patients. Of these, 50 patients underwent immediate repair of the partial mastectomy defect that included local tissue rearrangement in 14 patients, a breast reduction in 33 patients, and a latissimus dorsi myocutaneous or tho-racoepigastric skin flap in 3 patients. Nineteen patients had delayed reconstruction after radiation, of whom 6 had tissue rearrangement, 8 had a breast reduction, and 5 had a flap reconstruction. Positive margins were dem-

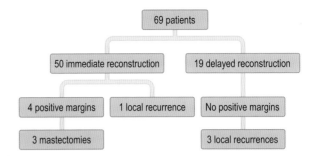

Figure 2.2

onstrated in 5% of patients and 75% of these underwent a completion mastectomy. Overall, 6% of patients developed a local recurrence over the mean follow-up time of 35 months (**Fig. 2.2**).

Considering the type of reconstruction, flap reconstruction had a recurrence rate of 13%. The authors suggest that perhaps these patients had larger tumors and larger defects and would have been better served by a mastectomy. The other forms of reconstruction had a recurrence rate of 5%.[8] The flap technique had a higher complication rate than tissue rearrangement and breast reduction in the immediate setting. In the delayed setting, the flap technique had a lower complication rate than the other two. These findings support what other series have shown. After radiation, a muscle flap is likely the best technique for deficit repair, whereas tissue remodeling is a better choice in the immediate or immediate delayed setting. Patient selection is important at all points in the process. The use of oncoplastic techniques encourages surgeons to perform larger-volume resections and the rate of positive margins in this and most series is acceptable if the patients with positive margins are willing to accept a subsequent mastectomy. Planning for delayed immediate reconstruction allows patients to undergo a re-excision of margins or to choose a mastectomy without loss of a flap and its associated morbidity.

The most recently published large series was from Italy by Rietjens et al, which compared itself to the NSABP B07 trial and the Institut Curie data by Clough et al, presented above. There were 148 patients who had breast conservation with oncoplastic technique and tissue remodeling, and 4 patients with a larger defect where a latissimus dorsi musculocutaneous flap or silicone gel implant was used. Concomitant contralateral side remodeling was performed in all patients. Again 1 cm macroscopic margins were obtained. The positive margin rate of 8% was similar to that observed in other series. All the positive margins were positive with DCIS. The local recurrence rate of 3% at 5 years compared favorably to the 9.4% reported by the Institut Curie and 14.3% in the NSABP trial. The authors concluded that for tumors less than 2 cm oncoplastic surgery can be considered as safe as mastectomy, and for tumors larger than 2 cm is considered safer than classic breast conservation. The factors most frequently associated with local recurrence were young age, positive margins, multicentric disease, and vascular invasion; however, none of these factors reached statistical significance. Only tumor size greater than 2 cm was statistically significant in the rates of local and distant recurrence.[9]

Asgeirsson et al performed a review of the literature for oncoplastic surgery. Their hypothesis in performing the review was that oncoplastic surgery would allow surgeons to feel comfortable in performing larger resections and reduce the incidence of margin involvement, as well as having a favorable cosmetic outcome.[10] Most of the series were small and reported a single surgeon's experience. Although these series show acceptable results, recommendations were made for a multi-institutional prospective trial, for longer oncologic follow-up and to establish criteria for more accurate patient selection.

Patient selection

Losken et al have developed a management algorithm for patients who are potential candidates for oncoplastic surgery. Breast size in relationship to tumor size is the initial criterion. Patients are divided into those who need volume replacement procedures such as a local or distant flap and those who qualify for a volume displacement procedure such as tissue remodeling or breast reduction. Volume replacement procedures are best performed in a delayed or immediate–delayed fashion. The advantages of a one-stage procedure are that it potentially avoids scar tissue, radiation changes and fibrosis, as well as a second trip to the operating room. The main disadvantage of a one-stage procedure when there is a positive margin noted on the final pathology report is that re-excision of a positive margin post-tissue rearrangement may not be accurate and mastectomy may be necessary.

The second consideration relates to the malignancy. Local recurrence is proportional to the size of the tumor and inversely proportional to the margin distance. In those patients chosen for immediate reconstruction, all attempts should be made to minimize the incidence of positive margins. This can be done through careful patient selection. Tumor size, location, and nodal status all play a role in decision making. The ideal candidate is one in whom the tumor can be excised within a breast reduction specimen and the patient is happy to have a smaller breast. It is most common to have DCIS rather than invasive tumor at the margins. In the series of Losken et al, all patients who failed re-excision of margins were under 40 years of age. It is those authors' recommendation that these two groups – those with extensive DCIS and those younger than 40 – be managed by a staged procedure.[11] When immediate reconstruction is desired, preoperative and intraoperative assessment of margins radiographically, macroscopically, cytologically, and pathologically should be performed. A generous resection, supplemented with cavity sampling and placement of clips to mark the original cavity, is recommended, especially in a one-stage procedure where re-excision of margins may be necessary.

Patient preference and satisfaction must be a factor in decision making. In a retrospective review of the NSABP B-06 data, postoperative evaluation of cosmesis was determined. Four groups evaluated the cosmesis: plastic surgeons, general surgeons, radiotherapists, and patients. Evaluation of cosmesis by the patient and radiotherapist was one grade above the surgeon and one or two grades above the plastic surgeon. Patient satisfaction was quite high and was based not on objective criteria (such as shape of the breast) but by success in retaining their original breast.[12]

Other studies have compared partial mastectomy to breast reconstruction post mastectomy in terms of psychosexual impact. Schover et al found that most of the differences in psychological impact of treatment appears to diminish after 1 year post surgery. Local treatment was not the crucial factor in psychosexual adjustment to the disease. There was no difference in level of sexual activity between the two groups. The authors concluded that if women are given medically appropriate treatment options and feel comfortable with their choices, the majority return to a good level of psychological and sexual functioning.[13]

The patient's psychological state is very important to keep in mind when selecting patients for oncoplastic surgery. Oncoplastic surgery is more complex and time consuming and so leads to longer operative times and longer recovery periods. For some patients the necessity of having multiple operations is daunting. Having positive margins after breast-conserving surgery, especially if done with oncoplastic techniques, is devastating. A patient who is strongly motivated to preserve her breast will better tolerate the uncertainty and the potentially more difficult process.

Summary

Certainly the field of oncoplastic surgery could benefit from a prospective randomized trial; however, until such a trial is complete, the continued follow-up and reporting of large series is helpful. Patient selection is perhaps the most important aspect dictating the success of oncoplastic surgery. Patients who require a muscle flap reconstruction are better served by delayed surgery once negative margins have been established. Younger patients and those with large DCIS components are also best served by the delayed–immediate approach. A patient should be counseled on the impact of oncoplastic surgery failure and possible mastectomy. In those patients having immediate reconstruction, all attempts should be made to minimize the risk of positive margins and complications that may delay subsequent treatment or lead to additional surgery. To reduce positive margins a careful preoperative assessment should be made with all available techniques, such as careful review of imaging, physical examination, and pathology. Thought should be given to the postoperative treatment that will be necessary, such as chemotherapy and radiation therapy. Intraoperatively, wide macroscopic resections should be obtained, intraoperative imaging of the specimen should be performed for improved orientation, especially when the mass is not palpable, and cavity margin sampling used as needed. If all these measures fail to result in clear margins postoperatively, a careful discussion with the patient must take place to decide whether an attempt at re-excision can be made safely and accurately or whether that patient is better served by a mastectomy. As the results of testing show in the long-term follow-up, patients derive satisfaction from all forms of local treatment if they have participated in the decision making.

References

1. Veronesi U, Cascinelli N, Mariani L, et al. Twenty-year follow-up of a randomized study comparing breast-conserving surgery with radical mastectomy for early breast cancer. N Engl J Med 2002; 347(16):1227–1232.

2. Veronesi U, Volterrani F, Luini A, et al. Quadrantectomy versus lumpectomy for small size breast cancer. Eur J Cancer 1990; 26(6):671–673.

3. Losken A, Schaefer TG, Carlson GW, et al. Immediate endoscopic latissimus dorsi flap: risk or benefit in reconstructing partial mastectomy defects. Ann Plast Surg 2004; 53(1):1–5.

4. Clough KB, Lewis JS, Couturaud B, et al. Oncoplastic techniques allow extensive resections for breast-conserving therapy of breast carcinomas. Ann Surg 2003; 237(1):26–34.

5. Renton SC, Gazet JC, Ford HT, et al. The importance of the resection margin in conservative surgery for breast cancer. Eur J Surg Oncol 1996; 22(1):17–22.

6. Tarone RE, Lipworth L, Young VL, et al. Breast reduction surgery and breast cancer risk: does reduction mammaplasty have a role in primary prevention strategies for women at high risk of breast cancer? Plast Reconstr Surg 2004; 113(7):2104–2110, 2111–2112.

7. Lehman CD, Gatsonis C, Kuhl CK, et al. MRI evaluation of the contralateral breast in women with recently diagnosed breast cancer. N Engl J Med 2007; 356(13):1295–1303.

8. Kronowitz SJ, Feledy JA, Hunt KK, et al. Determining the optimal approach to breast reconstruction after partial mastectomy. Plast Reconstr Surg 2006; 117(1):1–11, 12–14.

9. Rietjens M, Urban CA, Rey PC, et al. Long-term oncological results of breast conservative treatment with oncoplastic surgery. Breast 2007; 16(4):387–395.

10. Asgeirsson KS, Rasheed T, McCulley SJ, et al. Oncological and cosmetic outcomes of oncoplastic breast conserving surgery. Eur J Surg Oncol 2005; 31(8):817–823.

11. Losken A, Styblo TM, Carlson GW, et al. Management algorithm and outcome evaluation of partial mastectomy defects treated using reduction or mastopexy techniques. Ann Plast Surg 2007; 59(3):235–242.

12. Matory WE Jr, Wertheimer M, Fitzgerald TJ, et al. Aesthetic results following partial mastectomy and radiation therapy. Plast Reconstr Surg 1990; 85(5):739–746.

13. Schover LR, Yetman RJ, Tuason LJ, et al. Partial mastectomy and breast reconstruction: a comparison of their effects on psychosocial adjustment, body image, and sexuality. Cancer 1995; 75(1):54–64.

CHAPTER 3

Indications and Patient Selection for Oncoplastic Breast Surgery

Steven J Kronowitz

Introduction

The desire of many patients to preserve their breasts regardless of the cosmetic outcome has led to a more aggressive use of partial mastectomy, with more extensive local resections being classified in the category of partial mastectomy.[1] As partial mastectomies become more extensive, the risk of suboptimal cosmetic results from such resections is likely to increase.[2] In recent years, the proportion of breast cancer patients treated with partial mastectomy and radiation therapy (XRT) has increased. This approach is referred to as breast conservation therapy (BCT). This trend is due in part to increased mammographic screening, with a corresponding increase in the detection of early breast cancers. It is also due to the increasing use of preoperative chemotherapy in patients with large operable and locally advanced breast cancer, where significant clinical responses can allow for breast-preserving procedures in patients who would otherwise have required a mastectomy.[3-5] After BCT, 20–30% of patients are reported to have a poor cosmetic result, with deformities of the treated breast.[4-7] However, poor cosmetic outcomes after BCT are likely to be underestimated in the literature because many patients with poor outcomes are reluctant to seek further surgical treatment.

In this chapter, we present a management algorithm for repair of partial mastectomy defects based on clinically relevant parameters that should allow the clinician to better select the most appropriate patient indications for the various reparative surgical techniques.

Management algorithm for repair of partial mastectomy defects

It is well appreciated that most reconstructive breast procedures are based on principles and concepts, not on structured guidelines. The proposed management algorithm presented in **Fig. 3.1** has been designed to serve as a guide to assist in the decision-making process for repairing partial mastectomy defects. However, the final decision regarding the optimal approach is ultimately made by the multidisciplinary breast cancer treatment team and the patient.

Importance of timing of repair in relation to XRT

Waiting to repair a large partial mastectomy deformity until completion of whole-breast XRT usually necessitates the complex transfer of a large volume of autologous tissue. Patients who choose BCT often do so to limit the extent

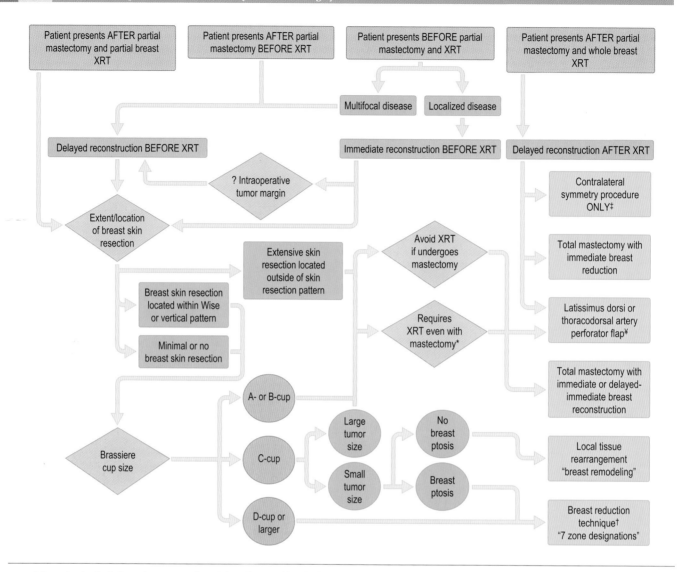

*   Scenario of patient who undergoes neoadjuvant chemotherapy with reduction of tumor size that becomes amenable to BCT, instead of mastectomy.
†   Prior to XRT, only perform the breast reduction on ipsilateral involved breast and then 6 months or later use the same pedicle design as used to repair the ipsilateral breast to perform the breast reduction for symmetry on the contralateral breast.
¥   Most applicable to patients with partial defects located in zone 6 or 7 of the breast.
‡   When performing a contralateral breast reduction for symmetry procedure only, allow for adequate time for the involved breast to achieve a steady-state in regards to volume prior to performing the procedure.

Figure 3.1   Management algorithm for repair of partial mastectomy defects. (Patient Presents After Partial Mastectomy and Partial Breast XRT.) This is an increasing group of patients who in the near future may become the largest presenting population for repair of partial mastectomy defects. In these patients, because the XRT was delivered only to the tumor site, the remainder of the breast parenchyma can be rearranged without the concerns of poor wound healing. Another advantage of this group is that a negative margin has already been obtained and the tumor cavity does not need to be elucidated (placement of surgical clips) for the radiation oncologist. The disadvantage is that an incision on the breast has already been made, which may interfere with the design of the skin resection pattern. The decision making with this group is based on the extent and location of the breast skin resection and the breast size. Patients with D cup sized breasts, or C cup sized breasts with small tumors, are excellent candidates for the breast reduction or breast-remodeling techniques. Patients with smaller-sized breasts will benefit most from a latissimus dorsi flap, especially since the XRT has already been delivered. It is unlikely that these smaller-breasted patients who only underwent partial breast irradiation will desire a completion mastectomy with immediate or delayed–immediate total breast reconstruction. (Patient Presents AFTER Partial Mastectomy BEFORE XRT.) This group presents both advantages and disadvantages to the reconstructive breast surgeon. The advantage is that these patients usually have already obtained a negative tumor margin. The disadvantage is that the specific location and extent of tumor resection are often not known. This is especially important in regard to determining whether the NAC has an adequate remaining blood supply from the underlying breast parenchyma. Patients who have undergone a central resection or by examination have evidence of sub-areola resection should have the blood supply to the NAC explored prior to committing to the breast reduction technique. Otherwise, the consideration for the best technique to repair a partial breast defect in these patients is also based on the location and extent of tumor resection as well as the breast size. (Patient Presents BEFORE Partial Mastectomy and XRT.) This situation represents the ideal scenario, incorporating the concept of the multidisciplinary approach in the care of the breast cancer patient. However, there are several important considerations in this patient population. Although most patients who undergo a partial mastectomy have localized disease, if a patient presents with multiple foci of disease the patient is probably better served with delayed repair because of their increased risk of a positive tumor margin or a severe breast deformity that would more likely benefit from a total mastectomy with an immediate or delayed–immediate breast reconstruction. The most important consideration in this patient group is the status of the tumor margin. The decision to proceed with an immediate repair or wait a week or two until a negative margin has been confirmed rests solely on the communication between the breast surgeon, the pathologist, and the reconstructive breast surgeon. Although it may seem intuitive to delay the repair until after of surgery and therefore they are not eager to undergo a major secondary reconstructive procedure. In addition, the difficulties associated with secondary repair within an irradiated surgical field limit the use of the adjacent irradiated breast tissue because of high complication rates. The use of prosthetic devices in this setting has been fraught with increased morbidity and is not usually recommended. With the increasing use of partial breast irradiation as an alternative to whole-breast irradiation, the use of the remaining breast tissue for reconstruction may become a viable option for these patients.

Delayed reconstruction after XRT usually requires a latissimus dorsi or thoracodorsal artery perforator flap; however, use of these flaps may increase the likelihood of arm lymphedema and may leave the patient without an autologous tissue option if further reconstruction is required in the future. At the MD Anderson Cancer Center, the role of local pedicle flaps in the repair of partial mastectomy defects has been changing. Although these flaps are still the most commonly used flaps for delayed repairs after XRT, they are now being used more frequently for immediate repairs before XRT (after confirmation of negative tumor margins). These flaps have been demonstrated to be useful in small and moderate-volume breasts and in patients who present with locally advanced breast cancer that will require XRT, whether they undergo a partial mastectomy (i.e., become eligible for BCT after neoadjuvant chemotherapy) or total mastectomy (**Fig. 3.2**).

In some patients who have completed XRT, a contralateral breast reduction alone, without repair of the involved breast, will improve breast symmetry. The advantage of this strategy is that the radiated breast is not operated on, thus eliminating the possibility for additional morbidity. The extent of the surgical procedure is limited and reasonable breast symmetry can be achieved.

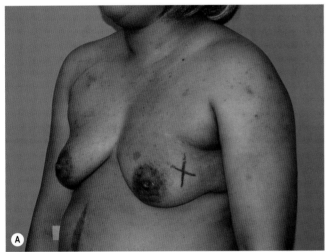 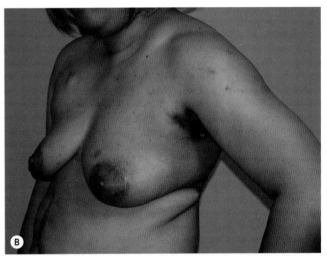

Figure 3.2 An example of a patient who would be a good candidate for an immediate repair before XRT with a latissimus dorsi or other local pedicled flaps is this 47-year-old woman who presented with a T2N2 tumor of the left breast, had an excellent response to neoadjuvant chemotherapy, and desired BCT. With C cup size breasts, she did not have enough remaining breast tissue after tumor resection to undergo the breast reduction technique, so she underwent immediate repair with a latissimus dorsi myocutaneous (de-epithelialized) flap. The patient had extensive scarring on her abdomen and, most importantly, was going to require XRT regardless of whether she had a partial or total mastectomy – an increasing group of patients who present with locally advanced breast cancer and then after neoadjuvant chemotherapy the tumors become amenable to partial mastectomy. **(A)** Preoperative view of the tumor located in the lateral aspect of the breast (denoted by black X). Because the patient had no involvement of the breast skin, the tumor resection was performed using only a periareolar and axillary incision. The latissimus flap was tunneled through the axillary incision onto the chest wall. The latissimus muscle was plicated to the shape and dimensions of the parenchymal defect and the skin island was de-epithelialized and positioned underlying the breast skin in the region of the defect so that, after atrophy of the latissimus muscle, contracture could be avoided and the volume in this region could be retained. **(B)** Postoperative view 2 months after surgery. Because of immediate reconstruction, the patient does not have the stigma of breast cancer surgery. If this patient would have repaired in a delayed fashion after XRT, she would have most likely required the skin island of the latissimus dorsi flap to be used to replace breast skin that frequently becomes deficient because of the contracted nature of the breast skin in the location of the unrepaired deformity.

confirmation of a negative tumor margin in every patient, many patients are at a low risk and would necessitate that they undergo additional surgery to perform the repair prior to XRT. After these issues have been addressed, further considerations in this group are also based upon the location and extent of skin resection and the breast size in relation to the tumor size. Patient presents AFTER partial mastectomy and whole-breast XRT. Unfortunately, currently this patient population tends to be the most common presenting to the reconstructive breast surgeon. The primary objective of this management algorithm and the techniques presented in this chapter is to eliminate this grouping. Although the decision making for this group is the most straightforward, these repairs usually require extensive reconstructive procedures that require the transfer of a flap. Although a flap provides its own blood supply to assist with healing within the irradiated operative field, its use to repair a partial breast deformity may hasten its use in the future, if additional reconstruction is required. The cosmetic outcomes of these more extensive procedures also tend to be less appealing because the skin of the flap does not match the remaining native breast skin. Attempting to repair a partial breast deformity after XRT using the remaining breast tissue is fraught with a very high complication rate. In some patients with significantly distorted breasts, it may be preferable to perform a completion mastectomy with an immediate breast reconstruction, rather than attempt a partial repair that will leave breast tissue that may be at risk of recurrent disease.

In the case of a severe breast deformity following BCT, the option of a completion mastectomy with total reconstruction is considered. The cosmetic outcomes of total breast reconstruction after BCT are less than optimal, primarily because of the relative inelasticity of the irradiated breast skin envelope and the increased risk of mastectomy skin flap necrosis.

At the MD Anderson Cancer Center, the most frequently used technique for repairing the partial mastectomy defect is to use local breast tissue. This is primarily because of the simplicity of these approaches and also because these techniques using local tissue will usually maintain the color and texture of the breast. If, however, an unexpected deformity results after partial mastectomy (**Fig. 3.3**) or the tumor margin status is unclear at the time of the partial mastectomy, consideration should still be given to performing the repair prior to XRT. In these circumstances, we prefer to use the remaining breast tissue for local reconstruction.

Although breast reduction is generally favored over local tissue rearrangement, the breast reduction technique is usually limited to patients with large breasts (D cup bra size or larger) (**Fig. 3.4**). Local tissue rearrangement can be a good alternative for patients with moderate-sized breasts (C cup bra size) who have minimal or no nipple ptosis, especially when the tumor is small, the partial defect is located in the outer quadrants of the breast, and involves minimal or no skin resection.

Immediate reparative techniques allow the plastic surgeon to participate in the planning of the surgical approach to tumor resection. Even if reconstruction is not required (because the defect is smaller than anticipated or the cancer is more extensive than anticipated and precludes partial mastectomy), the involvement of the plastic surgeon in preoperative planning simplifies any subsequent breast reconstruction that may be required.

Focality of disease

The decision to proceed with immediate repair of the partial mastectomy defect is dependent upon several factors. These include the results of preoperative imaging studies and intraoperative assessment. If there is evidence that the disease process is multicentric or even possibly multifocal, and the extirpative plan is to proceed with BCT, immediate repair of the partial mastectomy defect is usually discouraged. These patients are at high risk for a positive postoperative tumor margin. An alternative treatment in these situations is to delay the reconstruction and complete it prior to commencing radiation therapy.

Intraoperative tumor margin status

Attention to tumor margins prior to rearrangement of the breast parenchyma is critical. If there is concern during surgery regarding the adequacy of the tumor margins, the partial mastectomy wound is closed primarily without any tissue rearrangement. After confirmation of negative margins upon review of the permanent sections, repair of the partial breast deformity is performed. This usually is planned within several weeks following the partial mastectomy and usually does not delay the onset of XRT.

In our series,[6] only 5% of patients had positive tumor margins after undergoing immediate repair following partial mastectomy. This rate is lower than the positive

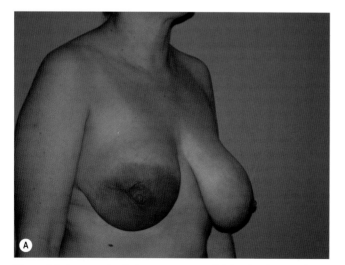
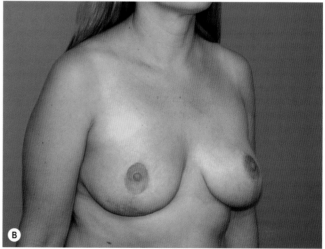

Figure 3.3 An example of when an unexpected deformity after partial mastectomy may require delayed repair prior to radiation therapy. **(A)** This 41-year-old woman presented 2 weeks after undergoing a partial mastectomy for a central quadrant tumor. The patient was very dissatisfied with the result and understood that the cosmetic outcome would be further adversely affected by the radiation therapy. Delayed repair before XRT was performed with the breast reduction technique. Because the extent and exact location of central resection could not be determined preoperatively – a disadvantage of delayed repair before XRT, the NAC was explored to determine if there was an adequate blood supply before the breast reduction technique was begun. The blood supply retained to the NAC was adequate for repair with an inferomedial dermoglandular pedicle. **(B)** Postoperative view 3 months after repair. The patient was happy with the result, as was the breast surgeon. Reproduced from Kronowitz SJ, Hunt KK, Kuerer HM, et al. Practical guidelines for repair of partial mastectomy defects using the breast reduction technique in patients undergoing breast conservation therapy. *Plast Reconstr Surg* 2007; 120:1–14.

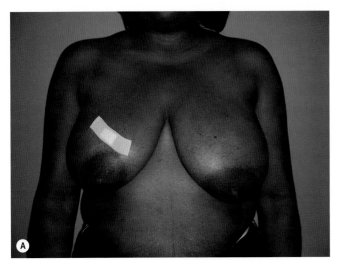 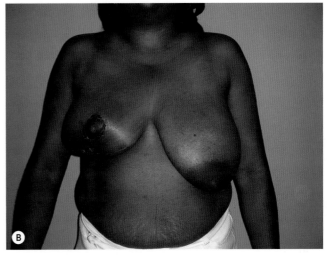

Figure 3.4 (A) A good candidate for immediate breast repair before XRT with breast reduction is this 41-year-old woman with a 38DD bra size who presented with a T2N0 (stage IIA) invasive ductal carcinoma in the upper inner quadrant of the right breast. She had localized disease with a single focus without associated microcalcifications. A Wise skin resection pattern was used and marked preoperatively in preparation for immediate repair with the breast reduction technique. The partial mastectomy was performed through an access incision along the superomedial limb of the Wise skin pattern so that after the repair there will be no stigma of breast cancer surgery. An inferomedial dermoglandular pedicle was used for the immediate repair of the defect. **(B)** Postoperative view 2 weeks after repair showing how the retained medial wedge of breast tissue filled the defect in the upper inner quadrant of the breast. As per our new protocol, the contralateral breast reduction will be performed approximately 6 months after the completion of XRT to allow adequate time for the repaired breast to achieve a stable form.

margin rates reported in patients who do not undergo repair[7] because the defect sizes in those patients are generally smaller. This finding of such a low rate of positive tumor margins should alleviate concerns regarding positive tumor margins after an immediate repair with the breast reduction techniques. Furthermore, our larger experience indicates that the majority of patients who are planned for repair because of larger anticipated defects will proceed to completion mastectomy with immediate breast reconstruction rather than additional re-excision.[6] The relatively low (5%) incidence of local recurrence of breast cancer[6] is further evidence in support of the role of immediate repair of partial mastectomy defects using the breast reduction technique as a definitive method of breast reconstruction.

Extent and location of the anticipated breast skin resection

It is essential to consider the anticipated size and location of the skin defect when choosing the most appropriate reparative technique. The need to remove breast skin during a partial mastectomy for invasive or in situ breast cancer is extremely rare and would only be indicated if the tumor was found to be within or extremely close to the breast skin. However, in the circumstance that breast skin resection (tumor extirpation) is required and located within the boundaries of the Wise pattern, the situation is ideal. When the skin to be resected is located outside the Wise pattern, it can be problematic. In such situations, consideration can be given to modifying the Wise skin pattern to incorporate the resected skin. If the skin to be resected involves only the re-excision of an existing

biopsy site and if there is an adequate skin bridge between the biopsy site and the Wise pattern, the biopsy site can be re-excised separately, and the tumor extirpation can be performed through an access incision located along the superior or inferior limbs of the Wise pattern (**Fig. 3.5**). Although the appropriateness of a separate access incision for tumor resection is up to the breast surgeon, this approach can result in an optimal cosmetic outcome with minimal distortion of the breast shape. When a large amount of skin excision is required to achieve an adequate margin, many of the advantages of BCT are lost. When breast skin defects are so extensive that they must be repaired using a flap, BCT may not be the best option with respect to breast reconstruction. Although a latissimus dorsi flap can replace a large region of skin, the differences in skin color and texture may produce a less desirable cosmetic outcome. Consideration should also be given to the volume status of the deformity and whether a latissimus dorsi flap alone will be able to adequately provide the necessary volume for the repair. In the event that a prosthetic device is considered, it may be preferable to perform a mastectomy with total breast reconstruction, since breast implants are often associated with additional morbidity in the setting of XRT.[8] In patients who are not candidates for a lower abdominal (transverse rectus abdominis myocutaneous, TRAM; deep inferior epigastric perforator, DIEP; or superficial inferior epigastric artery, SIEA) flap breast reconstruction (because of inadequate or excessive abdominal pannus, or abdominal scarring), a latissimus dorsi flap may be the only available autologous tissue source should the patient develop a local recurrence of breast cancer or a contour deformity after XRT.

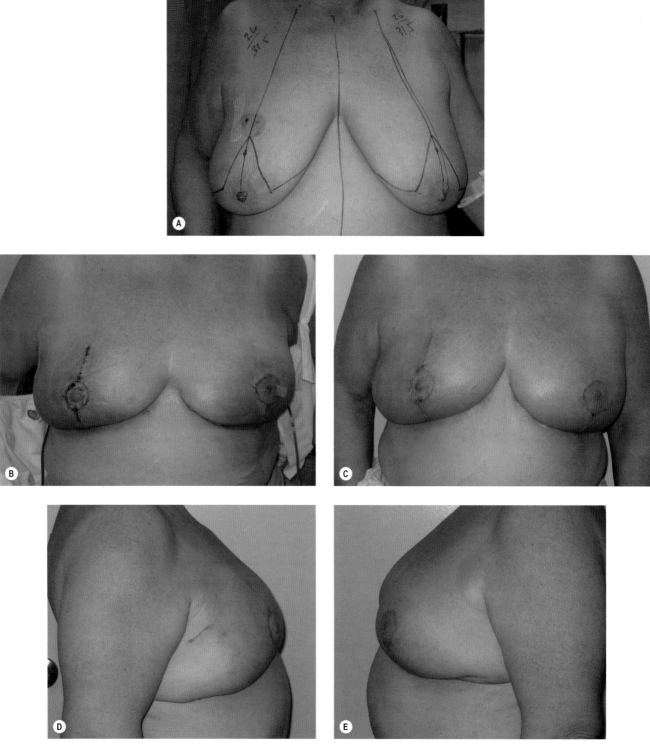

Figure 3.5 This is an example of a woman with moderate mammary hypertrophy with a right-sided breast cancer that is located outside the Wise pattern. In these cases the excision of additional skin can be made outside the pattern or the pattern can be adjusted to incorporate the tumor. **(A)** Preoperative image of a woman who will have a right partial mastectomy and bilateral reduction mammaplasty. It was decided to extend the vertical limb of the Wise pattern to perform the partial mastectomy. **(B)** Immediate postoperative view demonstrating the location of the skin incisions. The total resection volume was 440 g on the right and 420 g on the left. Drains were used for 1–2 days. **(C)** A 3-week postoperative view demonstrates good healing and excellent symmetry. **(D)** A right lateral view demonstrating natural contour. **(E)** A left lateral view demonstrating natural contour. Case provided by Maurice Nahabedian MD.

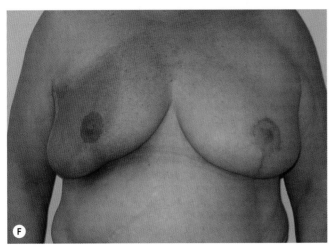
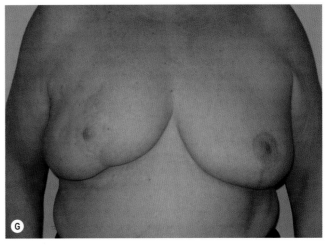

Figure 3.5, cont'd (F) A post-radiation photograph at 2 weeks demonstrating slight erythema around the right breast and a mild contour irregularity along the inframammary fold. **(G)** Two years following the radiation treatments. There has been no evidence of recurrence and the patient is pleased with the outcome.

Proximity of the breast parenchymal defect to the nipple–areola complex

Another important consideration in planning surgical management of breast cancer is the proximity of the anticipated breast parenchymal defect to the nipple–areola complex (NAC). When the anticipated defect is centrally located (sub-areola) within the breast, patients are advised preoperatively of the possibility that the only remaining blood supply to the NAC after resection will be from the skin attachments, which may preclude the use of the breast reduction technique. Other options include the breast reduction technique with a free nipple graft and local rearrangement of the surrounding breast parenchyma without repositioning of the NAC (local tissue rearrangement). Patients are advised that when the local tissue rearrangement technique is used and the cosmetic outcome is unacceptable, consideration is given to proceeding with a completion mastectomy with total breast reconstruction, thereby avoiding the adverse effects of XRT.

Impact of breast size and tumor size on repair

Most patients with an A or B cup breast size are not candidates for immediate repair following BCT surgery because the remaining breast tissue is usually inadequate to perform a repair, thereby requiring the use of a vascularized tissue flap to correct the deformity.[9] In these patients, along with some patients with C cup breast sizes who have large tumor sizes, it is usually preferable to perform a total mastectomy with immediate breast reconstruction to avoid the adverse effects of XRT. The radiation will sometimes distort the skin envelope of the breast and may result in an abnormal position of the NAC. Subsequent repair of these distortions is difficult to effect.[9] In addition, total mastectomy and immediate reconstruction may allow for the use of implant-based total breast reconstruction. This has been a relative contraindication in a radiated breast, especially in those patients who tend to have a paucity of autologous tissue options.

Although patients who have had a previous breast implant augmentation appear to have large breasts, most of these patients had A or B cup breast sizes prior to augmentation and therefore should be treated similarly to small-breasted patients.[9] Unfortunately, patients who undergo BCT without removal of the existing breast implant will often develop a severe infection requiring removal of the irradiated implant or a deformity of the breast with associated constricting pain secondary to capsular contracture with implant displacement.[9] Reconstructive options for these patients can be limited because of the XRT, which usually requires the use of an autologous tissue flap to assist healing. Many of these patients require a complex microsurgical procedure, such as a gluteal flap, because small-breasted patients tend to have minimal adipose tissue in their lower abdominal regions. An alternative for many of these patients is total mastectomy with removal of the implant along with immediate reconstruction. By avoiding XRT, they could be offered reconstructive options that include the use of a breast implant.[9]

In large-breasted patients (D cup breast size or larger) for whom partial mastectomy is predicted to result in a significant breast deformity, surgeons should consider incorporating immediate reparative techniques using breast reduction techniques. Patients who have C cup breast sizes, especially those patients with small tumor sizes, may also benefit from these techniques. However, C cup breast size patients with no nipple ptosis can be a difficult management problem[9] because they are not usually good candidates for the breast reduction technique. The lack of breast ptosis does not allow for any modification in the position of their NAC, which is why these patients can be more satisfactorily repaired using the local tissue rearrangement technique.

Radiation oncology considerations of immediate oncoplastic repair

Radiation therapy plays an important role in reducing breast recurrences and improving survival of patients treated with BCT. To date, there is no clinical evidence that immediate oncoplastic repair limits the effectiveness of radiation in achieving optimal outcomes. However, it is important that radiation oncology considerations are taken into account when deciding on the best approach for individual patients. Standard radiation treatments for patients treated with BCT include whole breast irradiation for 5–5.5 weeks, followed by a tumor bed boost for an additional 1–1.5 weeks. For the whole breast component of treatment, immediate repair often improves the breast geometry for radiation therapy and for women with large breast sizes may help to reduce acute skin morbidity. For the tumor bed boost component, however, the targeted tissue immediately adjacent to the tumor bed can be displaced and hard to localize. Accordingly, every effort should be made to mark the tumor bed region or keep it contained in a localized region of the breast. This can be planned with the treating radiation oncologist prior to the surgical procedure. Immediate oncoplastic repair should not be considered for patients who are going to be treated with postoperative partial breast irradiation. However, the increasing use of intraoperative partial breast irradiation may make immediate repair a more feasible option.

Summary

In patients undergoing a partial mastectomy, choosing the best method to repair the defect is essential in optimizing outcomes and minimizing the potential for postoperative complications. At MD Anderson, the clinicopathologic factors considered in the surgical decision making for reconstruction after partial mastectomy include the timing of reconstruction in relation to radiation therapy (XRT), status of the tumor margin, extent of breast skin resection, breast size, and whether the cosmetic outcome would be better after a total mastectomy with immediate breast reconstruction, thereby avoiding the need for XRT.

Most patients with medium or large breasts will likely benefit from immediate repair, whereas some patients with small breasts may not. Immediate repair of partial mastectomy defects is preferred with the use of the remaining local breast tissue (local tissue rearrangement or breast reduction techniques) because of the simplicity of these approaches and because techniques using local tissue maintain the color and texture of the breast. Waiting to repair a large partial mastectomy deformity until after whole-breast XRT usually necessitates a complex transfer of a large volume of autologous tissue, which many patients who undergo BCT are not willing to pursue. The use of lower abdominal flaps to repair partial breast defects is not usually recommended at our institution. Although the management algorithm presented in this chapter should prove useful, ultimately it is up to the multidisciplinary breast team and the patient to determine the best approach.

Conclusion

Ultimately, the decision-making process as to the best time to repair a partial mastectomy defect and the surgical technique to perform the repair needs to be determined on a case-by-case basis by the multidisciplinary breast team, along with the participation of the patient. The management algorithm presented in this chapter may serve as a valuable tool for the breast team to educate patients and to assist them in selecting the best approach for each patient.

References

1. Slavin SA, Love SM, Sadowsky NL. Reconstruction of the radiated partial mastectomy defect with autogenous tissues. Plast Reconstr Surg 1992; 90:854–865.
2. Clough KB, Cuminet J, Fitoussi A, et al. Cosmetic sequelae after conservative treatment for breast cancer: classification and results of surgical correction. Ann Plast Surg 1998; 41:471–481.
3. Cance WG, Carey LA, Calvo BF, et al. Long-term outcome of neoadjuvant therapy for locally advanced breast cancer. Ann Surg 2002; 236:295–302.
4. Shen J, Valero V, Buchholz T, et al. Effective local control and long-term survival in patients with T4 locally advanced breast cancer treated with breast conversation therapy. Ann Surg Oncol 2004; 11:854–860.
5. Chen AM, Meric-Bernstam F, Hunt KK, et al. Breast conservation after neoadjuvant chemotherapy: the MD Anderson Cancer Center Experience. J Clin Oncol 2004; 22:2303–2312.
6. Kronowitz SJ, Feledy JA, Hunt KK, et al. Determining the optimal approach to breast reconstruction after partial mastectomy. Plast Reconstr Surg 2006; 117:1–11.
7. Pawlik TM, Perry A, Strom EA, et al. Potential applicability of balloon catheter-based accelerated partial breast irradiation after conservative surgery for breast carcinoma. Cancer 2004; 100:490–498.
8. Spear SL, Onyewu C. Staged breast reconstruction with saline-filled implants in the irradiated breast: recent trends and therapeutic implications. Plast Reconstr Surg 2000; 105:930–942.
9. Kronowitz SJ, Hunt KK, Kuerer HM, et al. Practical guidelines for repair of partial mastectomy defects using the breast reduction technique in patients undergoing breast conservation therapy. Plast Reconstr Surg 2007; 120:1–14.

CHAPTER 4

Timing and Key Considerations in Reconstruction for Breast-Conserving Therapy

Elisabeth K Beahm

Introduction

In general, Stage I or II breast cancer can be comparably treated with either a partial mastectomy (lumpectomy, quandrantectomy, segmentectomy, etc.) followed by adjuvant radiation therapy – together referred to as *breast-conserving therapy* (BCT) – or mastectomy. Six prospective randomized trials have convincingly demonstrated that overall and disease-free survivals are similar between BCT and mastectomy (**Table 4.1**).[1-7] Historically, the limitation of BCT centered on concerns of a higher risk of tumor recurrence after BCT than following mastectomy for equivalent disease. While three of the previously noted six prospective trials demonstrated higher local recurrence rates with BCT, two of these studies showing higher recurrence rates with BCT did not have well-established negative margins, an imperative to avert recurrence (**Table 4.2**). Recurrence of breast cancer is complex and multi-factorial. Factors that contribute to recurrence after BCT (such as young age, lack of chemotherapy and aggressive disease) also predispose to recurrence after mastectomy. Recurrence relates not simply to the operative technique but to intrinsic tumor characteristics and the adjuvant and neoadjuvant therapies utilized. The Early Breast Cancer Trialists' Collaborative Group[8] demonstrated quite convincingly that the avoidance of local recurrence translates into a survival advantage and that, properly executed, BCT is oncologically equivalent to mastectomy.

Preservation of the breast is appealing to a number of women. The increased application of BCT in lieu of mastectomy reflects not only the demonstration of the oncologic parity of the technique in early breast cancer, but also a number of advances in complementary, parallel imaging and treatment modalities. Improved screening has resulted in increased detection of early-stage breast cancers. The use of adjuvant chemotherapy and endocrine therapies has lowered the risk of ipsilateral breast disease. Neoadjuvant chemotherapy has enabled some tumors initially too large to be treated with BCT to be downsized and rendered amenable to this treatment. These factors all have implications for determining the optimal oncologic result for women with breast cancer considering their treatment.

The interest in averting aesthetic deformity after BCT has increased as well, evidenced by the emergence of the discipline of Oncoplastic Surgery. The term *oncoplastic* is derived from the Greek *onco* meaning tumor, and *plastic*, meaning to mold, and combines oncologic principles with some form of local tissue rearrangement to avoid deformity with BCT.

Table 4.1 Survival comparisons for BCT and radiation versus mastectomy in prospective randomized trials

Trial	Endpoint	Number of patients	Overall survival (%)			Disease-free survival (%)		
			BCS + XRT	Mastectomy	P-value	BCS + XRT	Mastectomy	P-value
Milan[2]	18 years	701	65	65	NS			
Institut Gustave-Roussy[3]	15 years	179	73	65	0.19			
NSABP B-06[4]	12 years	1219	63	59	0.12	50	49	0.21
National Cancer Institute[5]	10 years	237	77	75	0.89	72	69	0.93
EORTC[6]	10 years	874	65	66	NS			
Danish Breast Cancer Group[7]	6 years	904	79	82	NS	70	66	NS

Table 4.2 Comparisons of local recurrence following breast conservative surgery and radiation or mastectomy in prospective randomized trials

Trial	Endpoint	BCS + XRT	Mastectomy	P-value
Milan[2]	Cumulative incidence at 18 years	7	4	NS
Institut Gustave-Roussy[3]	Cumulative incidence at 15 years	9	14	NS
NSABP B-06[4]	Cumulative incidence	10	8	
National Cancer Institute[5]	Crude incidence median follow-up of 10.1 years	19	6	0.01
EORTC[6]	Actuarial at 10 years	20	12	0.01
Danish Breast Cancer Group[7]	Crude incidence median follow-up of 3.3 years	3	4	NS

Optimizing outcomes

Assessing outcomes in breast reconstruction: BCT vs mastectomy?

Once the oncologic imperative is met, it then becomes incumbent upon surgeons to determine the best means to address reconstruction in breast cancer, incorporating aspects of patient satisfaction and aesthetic outcome. What factors will necessitate reconstruction in BCT? What are the most accurate determinants of whether local tissues or distant flaps will be the best reconstructive strategy? What is the appropriate timing of reconstruction in BCT: immediate or delayed? If delayed at what time frame is reconstruction most suitable? Can we pinpoint specific patient, tumor or treatment-related variables to guide clinical decision making toward the most favorable outcome? In this context, what factors should compel us to recommend a skin-sparing mastectomy (SSM) with reconstruction over BCT? While numerous studies have attempted to establish guidelines for optimal management in aesthetic outcomes in breast cancer, there is a lack of consensus.[9–21] In general, proponents of BCT and those of SSM with reconstruction have polarizing and opposing views. Preservation of the breast mound, skin and nipple–areolar complex (NAC) has been cited to afford a psychological advantage to BCT over mastectomy.[22–26] BCT additionally should avoid 'major' reconstructive surgery and the attendant potential for donor site morbidity in autologous reconstruction or implant-related complications such as fibrous capsular contracture, infection, and extrusion. In contrast, proponents of SSM with reconstruction would point out the excellent results currently achieved (**Fig. 4.1**) Free tissue transfer is considered the gold standard in terms of aesthetic outcome. It is durable and reliable (loss of free flaps for breast reconstruction is generally less than 2–5%). Implant-based reconstruction, while less natural in appearance and feel than autologous approaches, can provide reasonable results in suitable patients (**Figs 4.2** and **4.3**). Mastectomy for early-stage disease will generally obviate the need for radiation therapy and its untoward sequelae. The toxicity (both cutaneous and cardiopulmonary) associated with radiation in BCT is far less than that incurred with treatment protocols for advanced disease, yet it will limit reconstructive options, and the longitudinal effect on both native breast and flap tissues is difficult to predict.[26–30] Preservation of the NAC is considered an advantage in BCT, but the supportive data of the efficacy of this aspect of the technique are not clear. There are no well-defined outcomes studies on the retention of sensibility with BCT. The increased popularity of the NAC-sparing mastectomy, currently under prospective investigation at our institution, also may alter patient perspective on total mastectomy versus BCT (**Fig. 4.4**). Investigations comparing the aesthetic outcome of BCT versus total mastectomy with reconstruction have netted uniformly conflicting results.[2–20,22–30] Rendering

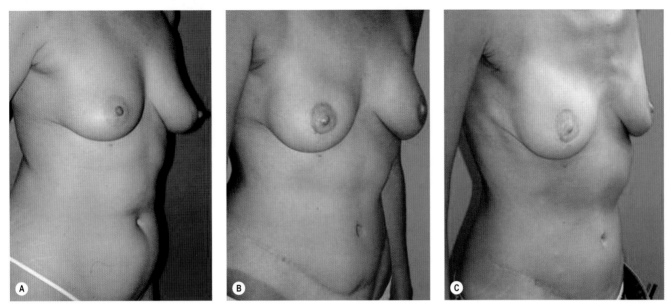

Figure 4.1 Results after SSM and free flap reconstruction. (**A**) Patient is seen preoperatively, (**B**) 5 years and (**C**) 9 years after bilateral SSM and immediate deep inferior epigastric perforator (DIEP) free flap reconstruction.

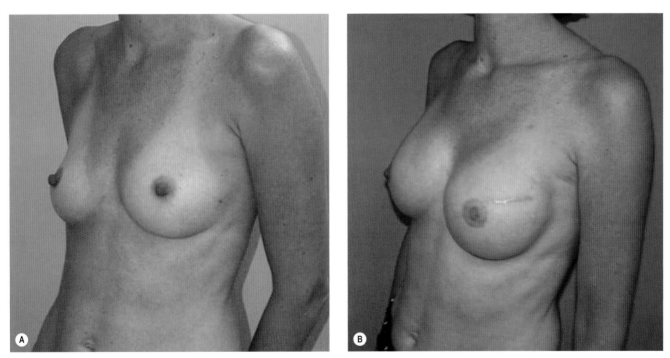

Figure 4.2 Results after SSM and implant reconstruction. Patient is seen preoperatively (**A**) and 3 years after (**B**) implant-based reconstruction and structural fat grafting after left breast cancer with contralateral augmentation for symmetry.

'objectivity' to aesthetic outcomes is highly problematic and dependent on a number of factors, including the patient's perception of outcome as well as the background and bias of the observer doing the ranking.[2–20,22–30] It is well established that there is poor concordance amongst physicians' assessments (plastic surgeons, radia-

tion oncologists, surgical oncologists) and patients' judgments in terms of aesthetic outcomes.[12,19,21,23,27,31] Resource allocation has taken on an increasingly high priority in the current medical marketplace. Cost analysis suggests that implant-based breast reconstructions are generally less expensive than autologous-based reconstructions

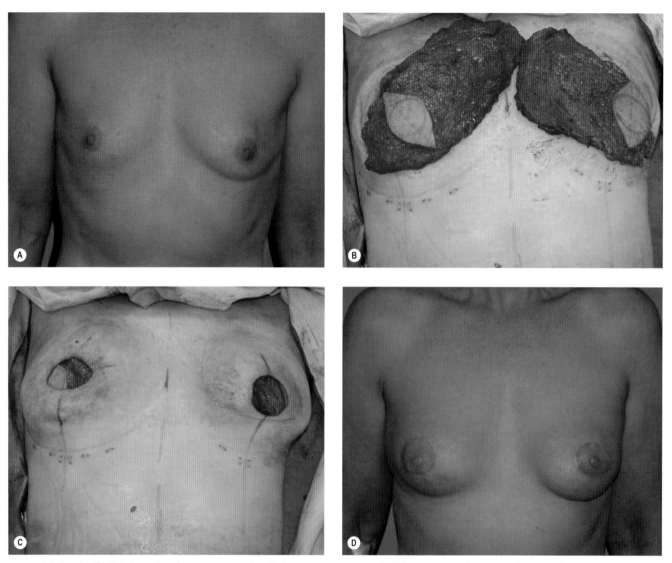

Figure 4.3 Results after latissimus dorsi breast reconstruction. Patient is seen preoperatively (**A**), intraoperatively (**B**, **C**), and 4 years after mastectomy and immediate bilateral latissimus dorsi and implant reconstruction for left breast cancer (**D**).

due to the increased operative commitment of the latter. The cost of radiation therapy renders the expenditure for BCT comparable to that of mastectomy with reconstruction.[32–35] In that vein, mastectomy alone with no reconstruction is the least expensive option, but few would argue that cost alone should be a deciding factor in determining such matters.[33] Patient quality of life and satisfaction after breast surgery are difficult to assess accurately in terms of the superiority of one treatment approach over another. Outcome studies have shown comparable satisfaction amongst patients undergoing BCT, mastectomy with reconstruction and even those with mastectomy alone without reconstruction.[2–20,22–30] There appears to be a complex interplay of variables,

including age, education, cancer fear, and premorbid psychological status, that contribute to patient satisfaction, making assessments problematic.[22–26] It is apparent from a number of studies that the perceived level of control that the patient has in the decision process of her treatment – both for the therapeutic and reconstructive approach in her breast cancer – is one of the most universal and significant factors dictating patient satisfaction.[22–26] While patients' decision making may be motivated by different factors to a variable degree, including preservation of the breast, cosmetic results, operative morbidity, treatment duration, and convenience, patients are more satisfied if they received the treatments that they wanted.[22–26]

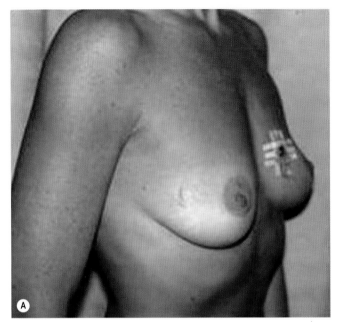
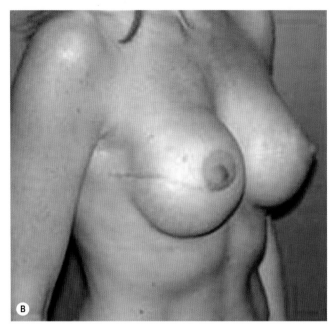

Figure 4.4 Nipple areolar complex (NAC)-sparing mastectomy and implant-based reconstruction. (**A**) preoperative view. (**B**) Patient with right breast ductal carcinoma in situ is seen 5 years after immediate reconstruction with saline implant and contralateral augmentation for symmetry.

Complications and side effects

Reconstruction in BCT: limitations of delayed repair

While patients may be happier with the treatment strategy they choose, this satisfaction is predicated on a favorable outcome. Poor outcomes should be anticipated and avoided as far possible.[22–26] It is estimated that 20–35% of patients treated with BCT have unfavorable outcomes, and a significant proportion of these patients are dissatisfied enough to seek additional corrective surgery.[9,10,12,16–21,31] Repair of a deformity after BCT is not straightforward. The effects of radiation therapy figure heavily in the complexity of effecting an adequate repair.[26–31] Prosthetic breast implants for repair after partial mastectomy are generally best avoided due to prohibitive rates of fibrous capsular contracture. Local tissue rearrangement of the index breast is limited by radiation.[36] Additionally, the patient may be asked to wait a significant amount of time (often 2–3 years after the end of radiation therapy) for the tissues to stabilize and the full effect of the deformity to be manifested prior to intervention.[37] Patients often find this longitudinal period of delay frustrating. Patients who initially desired 'less surgery' in their treatment choice for extirpation of their cancer are not eager for a significant operative venture to fix the problem.

The approach to repair of delayed defects after BCT, and the success of this operative venture, will vary by the extent of the deformity.[14–21,27] A classification of the deformities associated with BCT has been outlined by a number of authors, to help guide management and predict treatment outcome.[14–21,27] A straightforward system based on Clough[16,17] delineates deformity after BCT as: Type I (Mild) defects demonstrating volumetric deformity with asymmetry; Type II (Moderate) defects demonstrating contour deformity: Type III (Severe) defects with significant contour and volumetric deformity.[16,17] As the index breast is not deformed but smaller and usually 'perkier' than the contralateral breast, Type I defects are most commonly managed with a reduction mammaplasty of the non-treated breast, without manipulation of the index breast. This approach is the most straightforward but is predicated on the willingness of the patient to accept a smaller-volume breast and scars. The non-irradiated breast will invariably descend or drape over time, and a secondary 're-pexy' may be required. Fortunately, patient satisfaction with this approach is high (80%) and complications are limited (**Fig. 4.5**).[16,17] The more severe the defect, the higher the complication rate and the lower the level of patient satisfaction. Type II and III deformities usually require flap transfer for correction. The effects of radiation will compromise the aesthetic result and complicate the technical transfer and inset of the flap, and this must be stressed to the patients. Attention to both the skin and parenchymal deformity must be addressed, and due to the contracture in a delayed setting the defect will initially appear smaller. In order to avoid undercorrection, the original defect must be recreated and then the flap designed. The irradiated tissue will invariably contract over the flap and 'shrink wrap' around it, such that well-vascularized tissue needs to be introduced to all areas of the breast and chest wall and axilla, requiring correction to achieve the best possible result. The juncture of skin paddles between flap and native breast will usually have a color and texture mis-

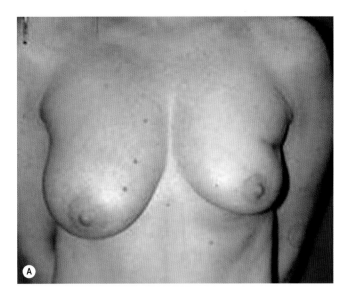

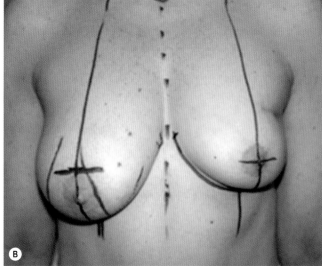

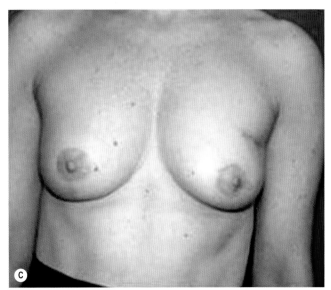

Figure 4.5 Delayed repair of mild (Type I) defect after BCT. The patient presented 2.5 years after BCT requesting improved symmetry with minimal operative intervention (**A**). As the index breast was generally well shaped apart from a superlateral contour defect, a breast reduction of the contralateral breast was utilized to improve symmetry (**B**). The 4-year postoperative result is noted (**C**). Figure used with permission from Boughey, Oncoplastic Surgery for Breast Cancer, Chapter 13, in *Textbook of Surgical Oncology*, Poston GJ, Beauchamp R, Ruers T, eds, Taylor & Francis, London and New York, 2008.

match and a contracted or biscuit/pincushion deformity (**Fig. 4.6**). The later contour deformity may be minimized with a more linear (as opposed to circular) flap design, but will be especially notable and essentially inevitable if there has been chronic inflammation or infection in the breast being repaired (**Fig. 4.7**).

Type II deformities may require a contralateral balancing procedure in addition to the flap transfer. Patient satisfaction with this repair at 3 years is approximately 45%. (Fig. 4.6).[16,17] Type III deformities will require a flap for correction, as well as a contralateral balancing procedure (Fig. 4.7). Patient satisfaction may be as low as 20% in this setting. A number of these patients may be better served by a total mastectomy and reconstruction, depending on the severity of the deformity.[14–21,27]

Avoiding deformity in BCT: key factors

As delayed repair appears largely unsatisfactory, it becomes clear that we must identify those patients who will likely experience a significant deformity after BCT and attempt to prevent this occurrence. The three factors that will reliably motivate a patient to seek reconstruction after partial mastectomy are: (1) volume discrepancy of greater than 20%; (2) contour deformity; (3) nipple malposition. While it is impossible to fully anticipate all unfavorable results, the aforementioned sequelae are the predictable result of several operative interventions in BCT. The most common causes of an unfavorable result in BCT include: (1) Removal of more than 15–20% of the breast parenchyma in a small-volume (A, B cup)

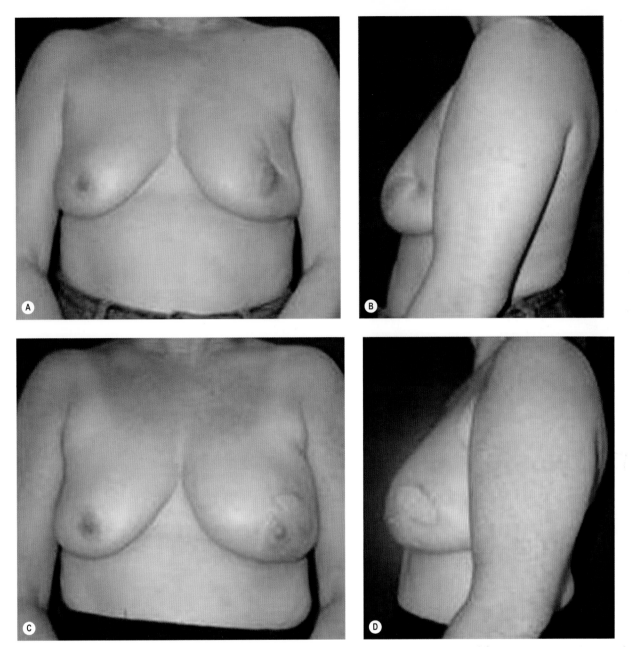

Figure 4.6 Delayed repair of a moderate (Type II) deformity after BCT. Defect demonstrates volumetric and contour deformity, prompting patient to seek correction (**A**, **B**). Ipsilateral pedicled latissimus flap was utilized to correct the deformity. Note the 'patchwork' appearance of the juncture of the latissimus flap and breast skin (**C**, **D**). Figure used with permission from Boughey, Oncoplastic Surgery for Breast Cancer, Chapter 13, in *Textbook of Surgical Oncology*, Poston GJ, Beauchamp R, Ruers T, eds, Taylor & Francis, London and New York, 2008.

breast or 30% or more of the breast in a larger breast. This volumetric discrepancy will be noted by and concern the patient. (2) Resection of tissue in an aesthetically sensitive area. Patients will often tolerate some contour deformity but not one in the critical cleavage area. Accordingly, a tumor extirpation that results in removal of a significant amount of parenchyma and/or skin, especially in an area in which there is a paucity of redundant tissue, such as the medial/superior pole of the breast, will likely be problematic in the long term. (3) A contour deformity will be made more severe if the focal defect results in adherence of the skin to the underlying pecto-

ralis muscle or fascia. These defects result when less than 1–2 cm of subcutaneous tissue is left on the skin flap and/or the parenchyma/fatty tissue of the breast is removed, exposing the pectoralis muscle/fascia. This defect is often manifest later in the postoperative course as the inevitable seroma (the result of dead space, and/or the intraoperative placement of fluid by the oncologic surgeon) resorbs over time. These deformities will be exacerbated by the longitudinal effects of radiation therapy. (4) Nipple–areolar malposition is difficult to camouflage. Removal of a relatively small amount of skin adjacent the NAC may result in nipple malposition. Even

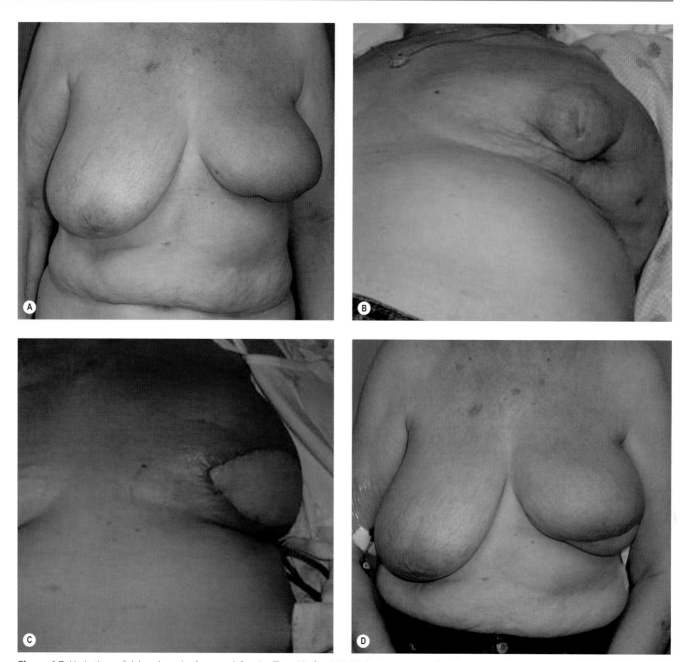

Figure 4.7 Limitations of delayed repair of severe deformity (Type III) after BCT. (**A**) Patient presented with a 14-month history of recurrent drainage from the nipple and abscesses refractory to conservative therapy and incision and drainage after BCT for T1N0 cancer (**A**, **B**). After serial debridement and intravenous antibiotics a latissimus dorsi flap was transferred and inset. The patient healed uneventfully, without recurrence of the infection, but was extremely dissatisfied with the color mismatch and pin-cushion deformity which resulted from the interface of the radiated, previously infected tissues and the non-radiated flap, despite meticulous intraoperative inset (**C**, **D**).

if little skin is removed, loss of breast parenchyma under the NAC will cause an angulation deformity or 'tip' the nipple. Excision of skin will both 'tip' and change the nipple position significantly. Excisions medial, lateral, superior but most commonly inferior to the nipple may result in a highly unfavorable deformity. This deformity is classically manifest after a transverse or 'Langer line' excision in the lower pole of the breast (between the NAC and inframammary fold (IMF)) and will result in severe nipple malposition unless a radial incision and/or some tissue rearrangement is employed and minimal parenchyma is excised.[9–21,27] These contour and shape deformities are not only visible unclothed, but often make it difficult for a patient to wear undergarments and certain types of clothing, prompting patients to request repair.

The parameters which appear to impact most significantly on the aesthetic outcome in BCT, and suggest the need for reconstruction with BCT or mastectomy with reconstruction, include the extent and location of the tumor and volume of resection, the ptosis and volume of preoperative breast size, and the ratio of tumor volume excised to breast size.[9-21,27] The most appropriate reconstructive strategy for management of these challenges depends not only on the characteristics of the defect, but also the willingness of the patient to accept a significant volume/shape change in the index as well as the contralateral breast to achieve symmetry, as well as their willingness to undergo a flap reconstruction. One of the greatest challenges in the assessment for the need for reconstruction in BCT is the accurate estimation of the impact of radiotherapy on the surgical defect. The balance of both treatment and patient-related factors will determine the reconstructive plan and timing, and ultimately which patients will be best served by partial mastectomy alone and those that will require reconstruction in conjunction with BCT. The approach must be further refined to determine those patients best managed with an ipsilateral tissue rearrangement, those that will necessitate both ipsilateral and contralateral surgical intervention for symmetry, and those patients in whom a regional flap may be needed and ultimately those in whom SSM and immediate breast reconstruction are preferable to BCT on aesthetic grounds.

Indications and contraindications

Indications for immediate reconstruction in BCT

Extent of resection and tumor variables

The absolute volume of the surgical specimen in BCT appears to be of less import than the ratio of the defect to the remaining breast parenchyma. Defects in large breasts are usually better tolerated than those in smaller breasts. In patients with a small breast, even a small defect can create a big problem.[9-21,31] This is especially important in tumors involving areas critical to the appearance of the breast, such as the medial superior pole, in which resection often results in a highly visible contour deformity or cases in which significant volume of breast parenchyma or skin between the NAC and IMF is resected, which may not only lead to a contour deformity but also a marked distortion of nipple position (**Fig. 4.8**). Unless there is a compensatory adjustment of both skin and parenchyma to correct for removal of breast tissue in these areas, contour deformities will develop and will be exacerbated by radiation. Immediate reconstruction is imperative in these cases as attempts at scar release in a delayed fashion are usually unsuccessful.[9-21,27-29]

The greater the extent of surgery, the more likely is deformity after BCT. In the breast, the defect incurred from resection is more accurately assessed as volume rather than weight, as the breast is conical in nature. The total breast volume can be estimated from a mammogram using the formula for a cone: $V = 1/3 \, \pi r^2 h$ (where h is the height of the breast off the chest wall and $2r$ is the diameter of the breast). Resection of less than

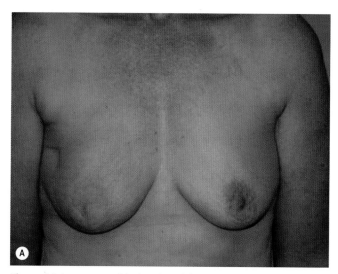
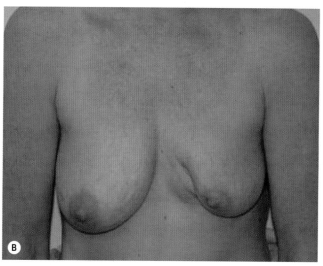

Figure 4.8 Importance of the location of the resection in determining outcome after BCT. Similar volumetric excisions demonstrate that a lateral contour deformity is far better tolerated and more likely to yield an acceptable outcome (**A**) than a comparable resection in the medial cleavage area of the breast. Resection in this area is likely to yield an unfavorable result and resultant deformity that will be poorly tolerated by the patient and should be averted with immediate reconstruction in BCT or consideration given to a mastectomy with reconstruction (**B**).

100 cm^3 results in better cosmesis than when larger volumes are resected.[14] Larger resections (120 cm^3) will usually require concurrent reconstruction to avoid deformity.

Additional factors found to contribute to a poor aesthetic outcome after BCT and necessitating consideration for reconstruction include inner as opposed to outer quadrant tumor location, need for re-excision for margin control, need for axillary lymph node dissection, greater extent of surgery, and existing significant volume discrepancy between the breasts when a tumor involves the smaller breast.[9–21] In these circumstances the surgeon must be critical as to whether the best result may be achieved by immediate reconstruction in BCT or conversion to SSM and reconstruction.

Patient-related indications for reconstruction in BCT

Older patients with more ptotic breasts have less favorable results after BCT, suggesting the need for immediate reconstruction or SSM and mastectomy. Obese patients and patients with large breasts are often excellent candidates for tumor resection in concert with bilateral reduction mammaplasty.[9–21,28,38,39] Obese patients present a reconstructive challenge after total mastectomy, as in the higher weight ranges (body mass index (BMI) > 35) patients may have significant morbidity with autologous breast reconstruction. Implants alone as a reconstructive strategy are rarely large enough to recreate a proportional breast for their body size and carry a high complication rate in this population. Breast reduction strategies can permit good aesthetic outcomes after resection of large volumes at any location in the breast. This approach is best undertaken at the time of tumor resection as local tissue rearrangement/reduction of a radiated breast is fraught with complications and not generally recommended. Additionally, reduction of the breast will often limit some of the skin toxicity and potential inhomogeneous dosing of radiotherapy associated with large, ptotic breasts.[10–14,27–29,36,37]

The prior augmentation mammaplasty patient presents a difficult management challenge in all types of breast reconstruction. These patients often have a high aesthetic standard and wish to minimize scarring and maintain their implants. The long-term sequela of implants that have been preserved in BCT is generally unfavorable.[9–14] These patients may be best served by mastectomy and reconstruction in order to optimize aesthetic outcome, but may be resistant to this approach. The larger the implant relative to the remaining breast parenchyma, the worse the result is after radiotherapy.[9–14] Patients must be prepared for the inevitable fibrous capsular contracture and distortion of the breast, as well as the potential for rib erosion and fractures and implant loss and infection (**Fig. 4.9**). Repair of these deformities will often require significant operative intervention with autologous tissue and patients must be made aware of the potential for these outcomes.

Radiotherapy: impact on reconstruction in BCT?

While the impact of radiation therapy on overall aesthetic outcome is, not unexpectedly, debated by surgeons and radiation oncologists, it is generally considered to be the single most significant obstacle in the achievement of an aesthetic outcome.[10–14,27–29,36,37] Irradiation of the breast usually results in shrinkage and fibrosis, with an average 10–20% decrease in breast volume.[26–30] Unfortunately, the degree to which radiation therapy impacts on the final result does not appear entirely predictable, and this makes anticipation of the need for reconstruction in BCT and/or the necessary degree of overcorrection of the deformity problematic. Patients respond to radiation differently, and patients with similar volumes of resection in breasts of similar size may have very different outcomes, depending on their idiosyncratic response to radiation. Certain factors have been more closely implicated in a poor result after radiation for BCT. Classically, application of radiotherapy to smaller breasts or more ptotic breast has been generally considered less favorable, and avoided, but this is far from universal. The use of a boost in radiation therapy, and/or therapy incorporating iridium as opposed to electrons, appears to be implicated in poorer results in BCT. Radiation following greater extent of surgery, such as significant undermining of the breast and/or devascularization of the breast as manifested by poor healing, skin flap compromise or fat necrosis also appears to be implicated in poorer results in BCT.[26–30] Mature breasts in which there is a lower volume of breast tissue and a greater degree of fat replacement tend to have a worse cosmetic outcome after radiation than dense breasts.[26–30] These criteria suggest the need for immediate reconstruction in BCT as correction of these sequelae is usually unsuccessful.

Perioperative history and considerations

Role of perioperative planning and neoadjuvant therapy in BCT outcomes

Limiting the volume of tissue resected will limit or potentially avoid any needed reconstructive effort and improve outcomes after BCT. Careful preoperative review of the imaging studies of the breast facilitates decision making regarding the appropriate localization technique (mammography or sonography), the number of needles to be placed for marking the extent of disease, and placement of the incision and therefore the precise area and volume to be resected. Centering the lesion in the partial mastectomy specimen will minimize the amount of normal tissue that must be resected to obtain a negative margin (**Fig. 4.10**). Patients with large primary tumors may benefit from neoadjuvant (preoperative) chemotherapy to shrink the tumor. In patients with tumors that are initially too large to permit BCT, neoadjuvant chemotherapy may make BCT possible, and has not compromised survival.

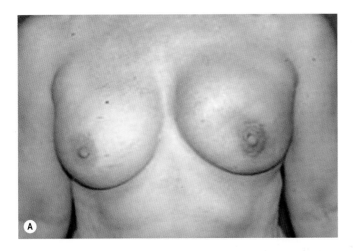

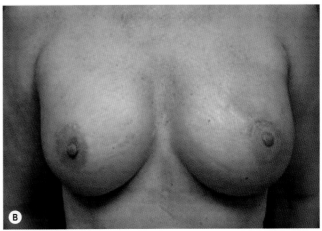

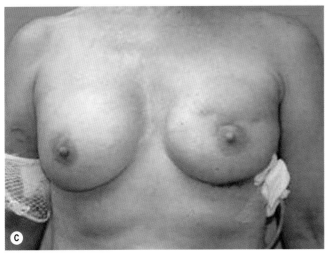

Figure 4.9 The sequelae of implants in BCT. (**A**) 56-year-old woman with prior silicone augmentation mammaplasty, presented 18 months after BCT to the left breast with complaints of a ruptured implant, pain and contracture. (**B**) Patient refused flap reconstruction and is seen 6 months after submuscular textured saline implant (**C**). Infection of left breast was noted 13 months after implant exchange, with recurrence of contracture. Implant was salvaged with explantation, continuous antibiotic irrigation and systemic antibiotic therapy.

In patients who are candidates for BCT at initial presentation, neoadjuvant chemotherapy may reduce the volume of tissue that has to be resected and thereby lead to improved cosmesis.[40]

Intraoperative margin assessment

Positive margins have been shown to be predictors of local recurrence and decreased disease-specific survival after BCT.[41] Aggressive local therapy is necessary to ensure adequate surgical margins and to minimize the risk of ipsilateral breast tumor recurrence. If immediate reconstruction is planned in BCT it is of course imperative that negative margins are verified prior to the reconstructive effort. The specimen must be oriented such that if re-excision is necessary the appropriate region can be easily identified and resection limited to the area of involvement. Accordingly, when immediate reconstruction is undertaken in BCT, extensive margin analysis is necessary prior to any tissue movement for reconstruction. At our institution we expend considerable time to assess the margins accurately. The specimen is inked with different colors to indicate superior, inferior, superficial, deep, medial, and lateral aspects and examined by the patholo-

gist. Specimen radiography is crucial to the intraoperative assessment of margins, especially in nonpalpable tumors. The specimen is serially sectioned, and reviewed by the radiologist and the pathologist. All microcalcifications and any marking clips placed preoperatively have been excised with the specimen. Only once the surgeon, pathologist, and radiologist are comfortable that margins are negative and all abnormalities have been excised should the tissue rearrangement for reconstruction in BCT begin. Surgical clips should be placed to delineate the territory of resection. These clips will guide treatment planning by the radiation oncologist.

Although intraoperative margin assessment can be time consuming and labor intensive, it is worthwhile, especially if tissue rearrangement is planned. Barrios et al showed that intraoperative evaluation of surgical margins by macroscopic, cytological, and histological analysis at the time of initial surgery revealed inadequate margins and led to re-excision in 37.3% of cases.[42] Intense intraoperative processing of the breast specimen as described above can significantly decrease the need for re-excision to achieve negative margins from 40% to 22% and can contribute to enhanced aesthetic results.[43]

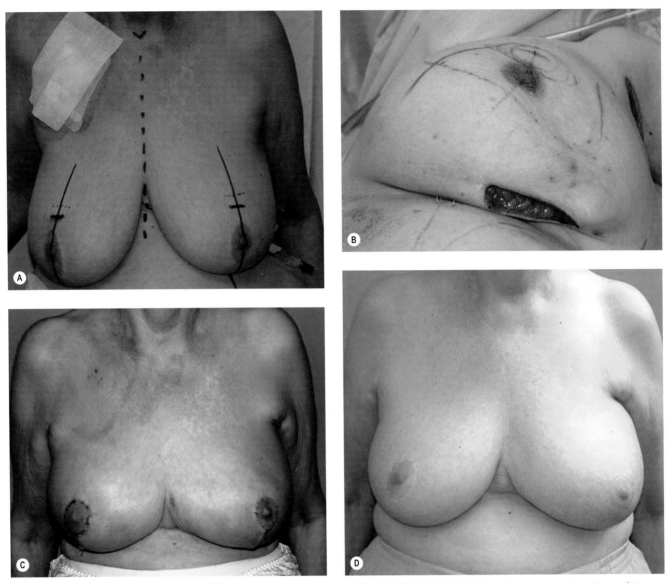

Figure 4.10 Role of intraoperative processing of the partial mastectomy specimen. The careful localization and processing minimizes the volume of tissue necessary for resection and therefore potential deformity in BCT and compromising surgical margins. Needle localization with a localization wire will precisely locate tumor, seen in situ, and the resultant specimen, in association with an immediate reduction mammaplasty approach for reconstruction (**A**, **B**). The short-term and 7-year postoperative results from a parenchymal pedicle approach utilizing a horizontal and vertical skin excision (**C**, **D**). Figure used in part and with permission from Boughey, Oncoplastic Surgery for Breast Cancer, Chapter 13, in *Textbook of Surgical Oncology*, Poston GJ, Beauchamp R, Ruers T, eds, Taylor & Francis, London and New York, 2008.

Operative approach

Surgical approaches for reconstruction in BCT: considerations for outcome and timing

Repair of defects resulting from partial mastectomy can generally be grouped into three main categories: local tissue rearrangement with composite breast flaps, reduction mammaplasty, and transfer of remote tissue in the form of a vascularized regional or distant flap. The technical nuances of these options will be discussed in subsequent chapters of this book. The following discussion will instead focus on considerations for the relative merits and limitations of each surgical approach and key considerations for the most suitable application of each reconstructive strategy.

Skin incisions

The unfavorable location and/or orientation of skin incisions have been linked to unfavorable outcomes in BCT.[9-21] In a small-volume resection, the skin incisions used for partial mastectomy have a significant impact on the aesthetic outcome of BCT. Oncologically, the scar should be centered over the tumor. Appropriate scar orientation may make the difference between a poor and an acceptable aesthetic result, and avert the need for significant reconstructive venture (**Fig. 4.11**). Oncologic surgeons have been taught to follow natural 'wrinkle lines' in the breast and to employ curvilinear incisions following Langer's lines (concentric lines parallel to the edge of the areola) or Kraissl's lines (natural horizontally oriented skin creases) in the breast. This approach can be problematic, as the majority of patients do not have significant rhytids in the breast in which to 'hide the scar' and the scar contracture coupled with underlying parenchymal loss results in noticeable distortion of the breast. Periareolar incisions are well tolerated, but only with small resections, and limit access for distant tumors. The

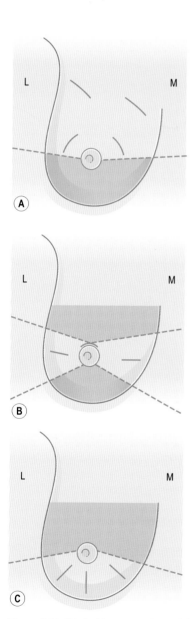

(A)

(B)

(C)

Figure 4.11 Skin incisions to minimize deformity in BCT. Periareolar incisions are most favorable, and curvilinear incisions will help minimize deformity in the more superior aspect of the breast, provided there is not a significant accompanying volumetric or skin resection (**A**). Radial excisions will minimize contour deformity (**B**), particularly in the lower pole (**C**). Figure used with permission from Boughey, *Oncoplastic Surgery for Breast Cancer*, Chapter 13, in *Textbook of Surgical Oncology*, Poston GJ, Beauchamp R, Ruers T, eds, Taylor & Francis, London and New York, 2008.

utilization of radial incisions is a far more favorable approach and is a fundamental tenet of reduction mammaplasty, adopted by oncoplastic surgery to avoid contour deformity and/or malposition of the nipple by complementary advancement of parenchyma and skin. It is imperative that skin incisions be planned such that if a mastectomy is ultimately required for margin control, the incision site can be comfortably included within the mastectomy skin island.

Local composite tissue rearrangement

Local tissue rearrangement is the most straightforward option for repair of partial mastectomy defects. This approach obviates donor site issues, preserves subsequent options for reconstruction and should be the first reconstructive strategy considered. Aesthetic outcomes with this approach are optimal when the defect is of limited size and the rearrangement is performed in the immediate setting. Composite breast flaps include full-thickness breast parenchyma plus skin and are best rotated or transposed en bloc. It is imperative to ensure that the tissues to be transferred are well vascularized, to avoid subsequent aesthetic compromise (or oncologic concerns) due to fat necrosis and scarring of the transferred breast parenchyma. These flaps, which were popularized by the late Stephen Kroll and others, are primarily used to effect a subaxillary shift of tissues from lateral to medial (**Fig. 4.12**).[17,44] Composite flaps assure a reliable vascular base and breast contour but are not appropriate for large defects, in which composite flaps can result in very noticeable scarring and distortion of the nipple. This limitation and the often extensive scarring attending this approach have likely led to its essential eclipse by reduction mammaplasty techniques for immediate reconstruction in BCT.

Reduction mammaplasty techniques

In women with macromastia, performing breast reduction in conjunction with the oncologic surgery permits BCT and can produce excellent cosmetic results. The reduction surgery permits better dosimetry and reduces the number of 'hot spots' and the volume of the lung and thoracic structures in the irradiation field. Reduction improves the homogeneity of radiation treatment in women with large breasts and lessens the risk of moderate to severe late radiation changes such as breast fibrosis.[26–30,38,39] Reduction mammaplasty also relieves symptomatic macromastia (shoulder grooving, cervical and thoracic strain, and mastodynia) and can be considered to improve breast health.[45] Other potential benefits of reduction mammaplasty for oncoplastic breast surgery are reduction in the risk of cancer of the contralateral breast. Although the efficacy of reduction mammaplasty as a risk reduction procedure is controversial, this premise has some support.[46,47] While the incidence of finding an occult cancer in a routine breast reduction specimen is low (0.16–0.5%), the risk may be higher when a

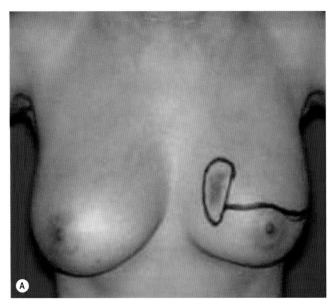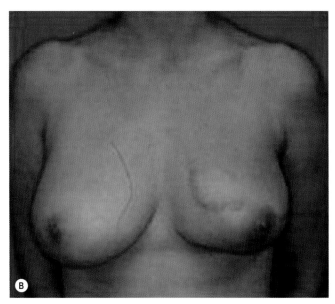

Figure 4.12 46-year-old woman 12 months after large superior composite rotation flap. Application of this technique in larger defects may result in volumetric asymmetry and nipple malposition. Case courtesy of the late Stephen Kroll.

contralateral breast cancer has already been diagnosed.[48] This highlights the need for bilateral diagnostic mammography prior to any surgical interventions.

When a reduction mammaplasty approach is being considered, the expected oncologic and aesthetic outcomes must be carefully considered. If there are concerns that the resection needed to obtain a negative margin will result in significant deformity that cannot be corrected with local options, reconstruction of the defect immediately with remote flaps or endorsement of a total mastectomy and reconstruction must be considered. These concerns are most common in small-breasted patients. Unless the patient has significant macromastia, resection of greater than 30% of the breast will usually result in an unattractive result. In the majority of patients with large breasts, this is not an issue as the volume of the partial mastectomy specimen is most often significantly smaller than the volume of tissue removed for breast reduction.

The effects of radiation on the breast after partial mastectomy are difficult to anticipate, and reduction mammaplasty is no exception. In the early postoperative setting, edema and residual seroma pockets give the breast a quite favorable appearance that may be different from the final outcome at 18–36 months after radiation therapy. Some authors suggest 'over-reducing' the contralateral breast to account for the likely fibrosis and shrinkage of the index breast in response to irradiation. However, this approach is not universally endorsed given the highly variable and unpredictable outcome of radiotherapy. The patient should be advised preoperatively that an additional small balancing procedure may be required on the nonirradiated contralateral breast. Breast reduction and adjustment of the irradiated breast have been reported but are associated with a high risk of complications and should be avoided. The reports of successful use of this approach noted poor wound healing, tissue loss, and nipple compromise.[36-38,49] Patients should be counseled that the success of intervention on a radiated breast, without the introduction of well vascularized tissue, will most likely not be successful.

In order to achieve the best possible aesthetic results of reduction mammaplasty, it is imperative to address the location and amount of both breast parenchyma and skin that is to be removed. To achieve symmetry, similar reduction techniques and scar placement should be used for the index breast and the contralateral breast. This may be difficult to predict preoperatively. Symmetry is most easily and often best achieved if the contralateral breast is shaped after the oncologic surgery on the index breast has been completed and margins verified. Flexibility in the application of an adequate vascular base for the breast mound in a reduction mammaplasty approach in BCT is critical and consideration for both skin and parenchymal components is important. The ultimate shape of the breast may be considered to result from the parenchyma as well as the skin. Short scar/vertical approaches are used in smaller, less ptotic breasts or a traditional inverted T scar in patients with significant skin redundancy (**Figs** 4.10 and **4.13**) The vascular pedicle for the breast mound can be adjusted to the tumor location, as nicely delineated by Losken[50] (**Fig. 4.14**). As tumors more commonly occur in the lateral quadrants, medially based pedicles, which derive their vascular supply from the internal mammary perforators, are very useful.

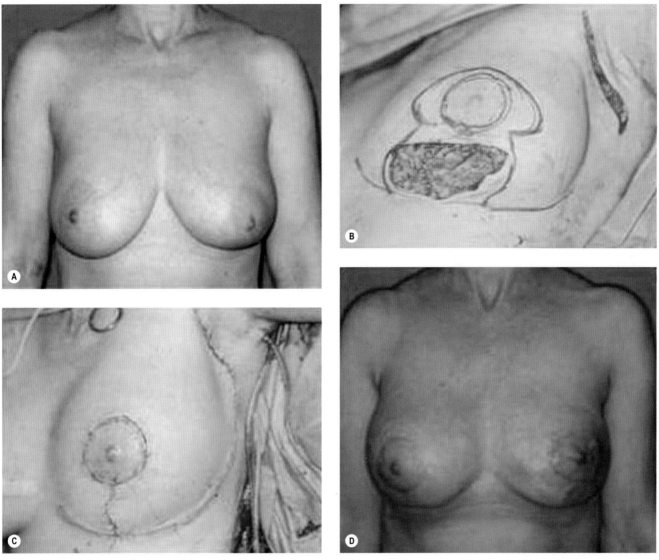

Figure 4.13 Immediate reduction mammaplasty approach with contralateral reduction for favorable result in BCT. Radial excision with advancement bilaterally lent to favorable outcome. (**A**) Preoperative view. (**B**) Skin pattern design and lower pole resection. (**C**) Immediate postoperative image. (**D**) 1-year postoperative view. Figure used with permission from Boughey, Oncoplastic Surgery for Breast Cancer, Chapter 13, in *Textbook of Surgical Oncology*, Poston GJ, Beauchamp R, Ruers T, eds, Taylor & Francis, London and New York, 2008.

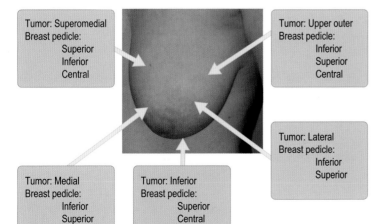

Tumor: Superomedial
Breast pedicle:
    Superior
    Inferior
    Central

Tumor: Upper outer
Breast pedicle:
    Inferior
    Superior
    Central

Tumor: Lateral
Breast pedicle:
    Inferior
    Superior

Tumor: Medial
Breast pedicle:
    Inferior
    Superior

Tumor: Inferior
Breast pedicle:
    Superior
    Central

Figure 4.14 The reduction mammaplasty approach for BCT. Vascular pedicle for the nipple and breast parenchyma may be varied depending on the location of the tumor. As most lesions are found in the upper outer quadrant this permits use of superior, medial and/or inferior pedicles in the majority of cases. Figure adapted from Losken[50] and used with permission from Boughey, Oncoplastic Surgery for Breast Cancer, Chapter 13, in *Textbook of Surgical Oncology*, Poston GJ, Beauchamp R, Ruers T, eds, Taylor & Francis, London and New York, 2008.

Successful reduction mammaplasty requires extensive and accurate intraoperative processing of margins. The need for re-excision because a positive margin is discovered on the final pathology review is not only oncologically significant but can seriously compromise the aesthetic outcome. Therefore, every attempt should be made to avoid the need for re-excision. In light of these considerations, it has been suggested that any manipulation of the contralateral breast reduction should be deferred until the final pathology review on the index breast is complete.[12,14,15,37–43,48] Most patients prefer to undergo immediate reduction of the contralateral breast to minimize the number of operative procedures, and this has been our standard approach except when there are extenuating circumstances. Patients must be counseled preoperatively that if there are questions about margin status or if the tumor is more extensive than initially suspected, contralateral breast reduction might be delayed or an alternate reconstructive approach might be needed. In cases in which margins are a concern – for example, in patients with large tumors managed with neoadjuvant chemotherapy – reduction mammaplasty can be performed after the final pathology review but prior to radiation therapy. As performing the mammaplasty as a separate procedure can delay the delivery of radiation, it is important to discuss this possibility with all members of the multidisciplinary breast team.

Regional and distant flaps in BCT

Regional or distant flaps can be used for oncoplastic breast surgery if the amount of breast tissue remaining after the oncologic resection is insufficient for tissue rearrangement. Autologous tissue provides an unparalleled match for the native breast, remains stable over time, and in some circumstances can obviate the need for significant contralateral breast surgery to achieve symmetry. In patients with an established breast deformity after BCT, vascularized autologous flaps are the mainstay for re-establishment of a normal breast form because of the extraordinarily high complication rate of implant-based reconstruction of irradiated breasts. In the setting of partial breast reconstruction, these advantages must be balanced with the potential limitations of vascularized flaps, which primarily relate to the donor site and may include contour deformity, pain, dysesthesias, and even hernia formation as well as the effect of radiotherapy. Additionally, it must be remembered that repair of a partial mastectomy defect with autologous tissue may significantly limit the patient's future options for breast reconstruction in case of recurrence.

Latissimus dorsi and thoracodorsal artery perforator flaps

The latissimus dorsi (LD) flap, based on the thoracodorsal vessels, has long been a mainstay of breast reconstruction after partial mastectomy (see Figs 4.6 and 4.7). The LD flap is robust, reliable, can be harvested with or without a skin paddle, and the anatomy is well studied.[51] Latissimus flaps are particularly helpful for lateral defects, superior defects and in small breasts, where local rearrangement is limited and even a relatively small-volume resection may result in distortion of the nipple position and loss of breast contour and volume. The flap has a more limited application in very medial defects due to limitations of pedicle length in many patients.

Immediate repair of a BCT defect with the LD flap is technically easier, is associated with a lower complication rate, and potentially involves fewer operative steps compared with delayed repair (**Fig. 4.15**).[52] The difficulty with the immediate approach is that it is difficult to predict the degree of LD muscle atrophy and the impact of radiation therapy on breast volume and shape, which in turn makes it difficult to determine the degree of correction necessary. Most practitioners overcorrect the defect by 10–25% in an effort to compensate for LD muscle atrophy and the effects of radiation, but this approach is imprecise.

The donor site of the myocutaneous LD flap can be aesthetically problematic, especially if a significant amount of skin is needed for the breast. The anticipated location and extent of the scar as well as the longevity of postoperative drains to minimize seroma formation should be thoroughly vetted with the patient (Fig. 4.15). A muscle-only flap, transferred via endoscopic or endoscopic-assisted harvest, will provide a far more favorable donor site in terms of scar and seroma accumulation. Traditional LD myocutaneous flaps with or without skin sacrifice a functional muscle, and the impact of muscle harvest on shoulder function is not entirely clear. Early reports suggested that there was little or no functional loss with muscle harvest, while some recent studies suggest a negative impact of LD muscle harvest on the activities of daily living in a certain proportion of patients. Accordingly, LD muscle sacrifice is not suggested in patients heavily reliant on their shoulder girdle strength, such as patients who have to use crutches.

Several modifications of the LD muscle flap have been proposed to minimize the functional impact on the donor site, including the 'split' LD flap described by Tobin[53] and, more recently, LD 'mini' flaps. In these modifications, the LD muscle is split along the vascular axis utilizing either the descending (vertical) branch or the transverse (horizontal) branch of the thoracodorsal artery. The most recent evolution of the LD flap is the thoracodorsal artery perforator (TAP) flap, in which no muscle or only a very small amount of muscle is harvested.[54,55]

The TAP flap is based on one of the two to three cutaneous perforators off the vertical thoracodorsal artery. The proximal perforator pierces the muscle and enters the subcutaneous tissue approximately 8 cm below the posterior axillary fold and 2–3 cm posterior to the lateral border of the muscle; a second perforator is usually present 2–4 cm distal to the first (**Fig. 4.16**). The TAP flap represents the current evolution in reconstructive surgery

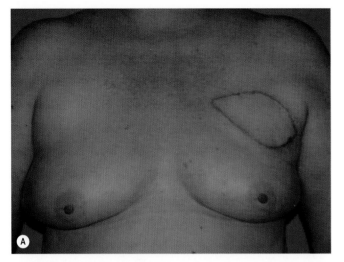

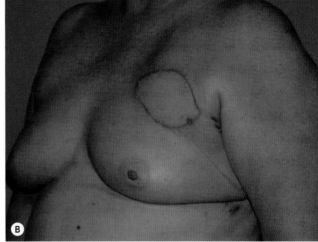

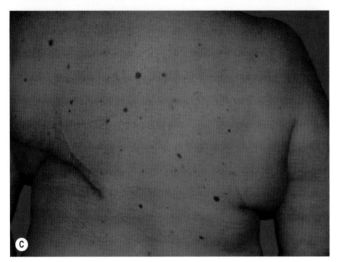

Figure 4.15 Immediate repair of large skin and parenchymal defect with latissimus dorsi (LD) myocutaneous flap. The patient wished to maintain her nipple and her breast volume. The superior location of the lesion and the large size of the defect (30% of the breast) precluded adequate reconstruction without the introduction of well-vascularized tissue. Flap was overcorrected by approximately 20%. Patient is seen 10 months after the end of radiation therapy. Note the improved outcome and contour of the LD flap breast interface in this immediate reconstruction compared to the delayed attempts at repair (see Figs 4.6 and 4.7). In addition to persistent seroma, the aesthetics of the back donor site may be a significant aesthetic consideration in a myocutaneous LD flap with a large skin paddle that is unfavorably located.

towards flap designs that reduce donor site deformity through flap harvest in which the perforating vessels are dissected free from the surrounding muscle and left in the donor site.[54,55] This approach is technically complex, subject to anatomic variations, and requires an experienced surgeon. The utility of TAP flaps for delayed reconstruction after BCT after irradiation remains unclear and awaits further study. In this setting, a traditional myocutaneous LD flap may be the safest option for repair of partial mastectomy defects.

Intercostal artery perforator flap

The intercostal artery perforator (ICAP) flap evolved from the thoracoepigastric flap, which was one of the first flaps used in breast reconstruction. The ICAP flap is based on a perforator found anterior to the LD muscle border and can be harvested without any compromise of the thoracodorsal vessels. The intercostal vessels are dissected to their origin through a split serratus anterior muscle, and may be rendered sensate. The vascular pedicle is short (4–5 cm), and the ICAP flap is best utilized for small lateral defects. While the pedicle can be extended with

dissection along the rib margin, this is difficult and may compromise the integrity of the vascular pedicle. The cutaneous territory of this flap is not well studied and awaits further delineation. Currently this flap appears to be most suited to repair of small, favorably oriented BCT defects in an immediate setting.[55]

Distant flaps in partial mastectomy

A number of distant flaps are potentially available for reconstruction of the partial mastectomy defect, including those from the abdomen, buttocks, and thighs. Vascularized flaps from the lower abdominal wall have emerged as the gold standard for breast reconstruction after mastectomy. The lower abdominal territory provides an unparalleled volume of high-quality skin and subcutaneous tissue for reconstruction, and a variety of potential vascular pedicles from the deep and superficial epigastric systems. The transverse rectus abdominis myocutaneous (TRAM) flap, based on the deep system, remains the autologous flap most commonly used for total breast reconstruction, but has been refined to improve the vascularity of the flap and minimize abdomi-

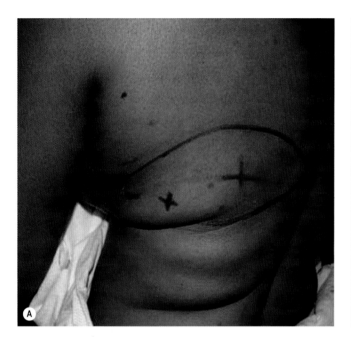

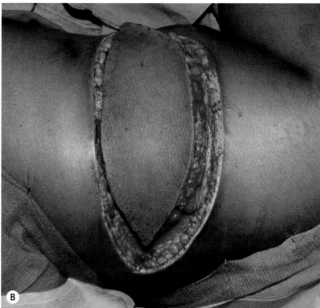

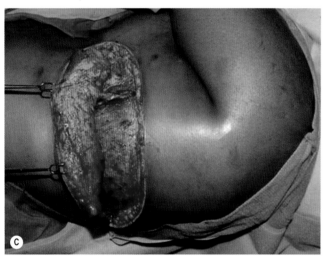

Figure 4.16 Thoracodorsal perforator (TAP) flap. The TAP flap is based on one of the two to three cutaneous perforators off the vertical thoracodorsal artery. (**A**) The perforators are localized preoperatively with a Doppler. The proximal perforator pierces the muscle and enters the subcutaneous tissue approximately 8 cm below the posterior axillary fold. (**B**, **C**) This permits transfer of a large amount of skin and subcutaneous tissue without the need to sacrifice muscle. Owing to pedicle limitations the reach of this flap is limited to lateral defects of the breast, but application is increasing with experience utilizing the flap.

nal donor site morbidity, with variants of free and perforator flap configurations. These flaps can and have reliably been used to correct a deformity after BCT, but it remains unclear whether this is appropriate (**Fig. 4.17**). The utilization of a large distant flap for partial breast reconstruction is controversial. While distant flaps are reliable, they are a significant reconstructive venture and carry potential donor morbidity, including scarring, contour deformity, pain, and abdominal hernia or bulge. More importantly, the oncologic integrity of this application is problematic, most particularly in an immediate setting. In the event of immediate flap transfer and a positive margin, the flap would need to be sacrificed. In the event of tumor recurrence after BCT, if a distant flap had been utilized previously the best option for repair of a total mastectomy would be unavailable (**Fig. 4.18**). The other concern in

utilizing a flap for immediate reconstruction in BCT is the effect of radiation on the flap. In cases of total mastectomy it is generally advised to delay reconstruction with a flap until after radiation therapy, due to the untoward and unpredictable effects on the flap, which may result in significant fibrosis and shrinkage. Accordingly, the utilization of a distant flap immediately is imprudent. The issue of delayed reconstruction with a distant flap is technically more challenging, but oncologically more tenable. While the incidence of a true recurrence or second primary after BCT compared to mastectomy is controversial, it does still remain an issue and an appropriate time frame for clearance by oncology is imperative. Patients must be informed of their options and considered for a completion mastectomy with flap reconstruction in lieu of delayed repair of a partial defect.

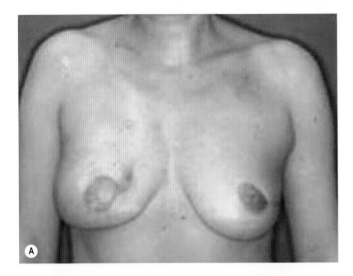

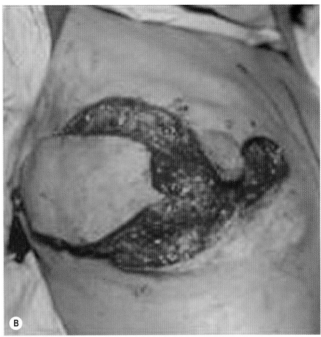

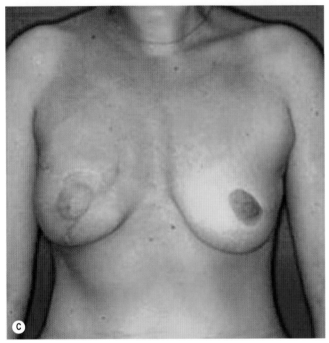

Figure 4.17 (**A**) 57-year-old woman with positive positive margins after partial breast excision. The patient wished to maintain breast volume and nipple, due to size of skin and parenchymal defect. (**B**) A free transverse rectus myocutaneous (TRAM) flap was transferred and revascularized to the thoracodorsal vessels. (**C**) The patient is seen 10 months postoperatively. Case courtesy of the late Stephen Kroll.

Implants after partial mastectomy

The use of implants for correction of partial mastectomy defects is fraught with significant short-term and long-term complications. Implant loss and fibrous capsular contracture with pain and distortion of the breast may occur, and the aesthetic outcomes are generally considered to be poor, and even worse than those of previously augmented women who subsequently undergo BCT.[56] True assessment of the complication rate and outcomes with implants is particularly difficult because of the retrospective nature of the studies published to date, use of subjective, non-standardized measures of outcome, short follow-up and small study size. We do not advise the use of implants for either immediate or delayed defect repair associated with partial mastectomy.

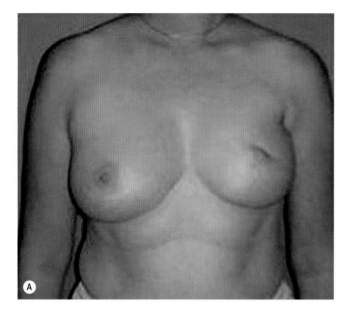

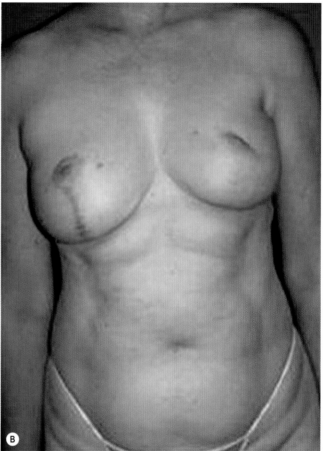

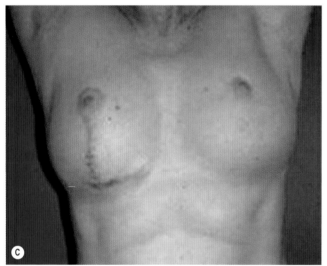

Figure 4.18 Recurrence after partial mastectomy. (**A**) The patient underwent BCT of the left breast with a result volumetric and nipple asymmetry and deformity. (**B**, **C**) Three years following treatment she desired correction of the defect. She refused flap reconstruction and underwent a contralateral balancing procedure. Six months following this procedure she developed a recurrent cancer in the index breast, necessitating mastectomy and flap reconstruction. (**D**) Patient is seen 12 months after transfer of a unilateral deep inferior epigastric perforator flap. She refused nipple–areolar reconstruction. Figure used with permission from Boughey, Oncoplastic Surgery for Breast Cancer, Chapter 13, in *Textbook of Surgical Oncology*, Poston GJ, Beauchamp R, Ruers T, eds, Taylor & Francis, London and New York, 2008.

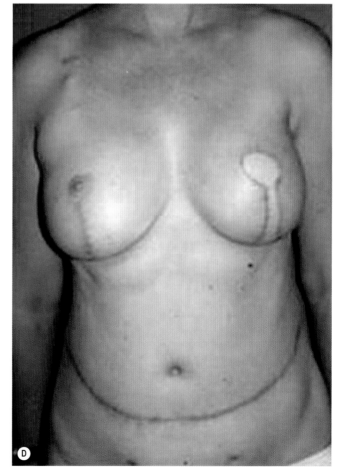

Future considerations: structural fat grafting

The application of free fat grafting in the breast appears to hold significant promise, particularly in the correction of small, isolated contour deformities. Several recent reports have demonstrated the efficacy of autologous fat grafting in both reconstructive and aesthetic applications using small aliquots of fat delivered through multiple passes through the tissues. Encouraging reports of improvement (softening) of radiated tissues following fat grafting have prompted the speculation of a 'stem cell' mediated process.[57,58] The clinical efficacy of this technique in cases of breast reconstruction has been empirically presented.[5,58] While this procedure would seem especially encouraging for the delayed correction of partial mastectomy defects, the ultimate fate of the fat grafts, their quantification in vivo, and their mechanism of action on the surrounding biologic milieu are currently unknown. Previously considered ineffective and even dangerous, further prospective, controlled studies are warranted to further delineate the effects of fat grafting prior to the widespread application of this technique in a native female breast under surveillance.

Partial mastectomy: guiding principles for reconstructive options and timing

The decision to undertake a partial mastectomy, or instead endorse a total mastectomy for breast cancer, is ultimately an oncologic determination. In those cases in which these two treatment options are oncologically equivalent, patients need to participate in the decision-making process in order to maximize their sense of satisfaction with their treatment outcomes. Measures of satisfaction and quality of life after various approaches to breast cancer treatment and reconstruction are highly problematic to assess. Patients' satisfaction in reconstructive breast surgery may fade as they become more temporally detached from the acute management of their cancer, and less satisfied with the appearance of the breast. In obese and macromastic patients a reduction approach for immediate reconstruction in conjunction with the partial mastectomy is often the most efficacious means of managing breast reconstruction. These patients are poor candidates for traditional autologous and prosthetic means of breast reconstruction after total mastectomy. In thinner patients, while retention of the breast is appealing, the realistic aesthetic sequelae of resection of a large portion of the breast must be taken into account. The primary factors prompting patients to seek delayed reconstruction after partial mastectomy are NAC malposition, contour deformity, and significant volume discrepancy. In general, these defects can be anticipated and should be avoided by immediate reconstruction of the partial mastectomy, or conversion to an SSM and reconstruction. Resection of greater than 20–30% of the breast, unless the patient has true macromastia, will usually result in a defect that is unattractive and may be better managed with mastectomy and reconstruction. These limitations are particularly important in small-breasted women, in which a relatively small volume defect (15–20%) may have significant implications. Accordingly, it appears better to consider options in small and large-breasted women separately. Tumor location, regardless of breast size, may also be a significant factor in terms of outcome. Resection of a tumor under the NAC and/or between the NAC and inframammary fold and those with a significant superomedial component must be managed very carefully to avoid a significant NAC distortion and contour deformity. Unless there is a compensatory adjustment of skin and parenchyma to correct these deficient areas, contour deformities, which may not be manifest in the immediate postoperative period when they are masked by edema and seroma, will develop, persist and be exacerbated by radiation. The importance of considering the necessity of immediate reconstruction after BCT is important as the ability to correct these deformities in a secondary fashion is limited, technically challenging and usually deemed unsatisfactory by patients. Radiation, which is vital to the application of breast-conserving surgery, greatly impacts upon the feasibility and technical aspects of ultimately rendering an aesthetic breast. Timing in delayed reconstruction of partial mastectomy defects is problematic. Edema in the radiated breast takes an extended period of time to fully settle; some authors have recommended waiting 3 years after therapy before attempting correction, but there are no hard data to this effect. Reconstruction of the radiated breast will generally require flap reconstruction. Local tissue rearrangement in the radiated breast is risky and rarely successful. Even the introduction of well-vascularized tissues unsullied by radiation will not usually fully correct the deformity owing to the enhanced scarring from the surrounding radiated bed. Radiation permanently affects the fibroblast DNA which exacerbates scarring and fibrosis. Patients must be made aware of the limitations that radiation poses on long-term reconstructive options. The possibility of local recurrence or a second primary following partial mastectomy and radiation must be considered. Reconstruction in this setting is problematic and will necessitate a vascularized flap. As such, in patients with a paucity of autologous donor sites we suggest the use of local options for immediate reconstruction of the partial mastectomy defect such as local tissue rearrangement or reduction approaches. If the breast defect is beyond the scope of these techniques, conversion to a mastectomy with reconstruction is preferable (**Figs 4.19** and **4.20**). Medical oncology, radiation therapy, surgical oncology and plastic surgery must work together with a multidisciplinary approach to help guide patient decisions.

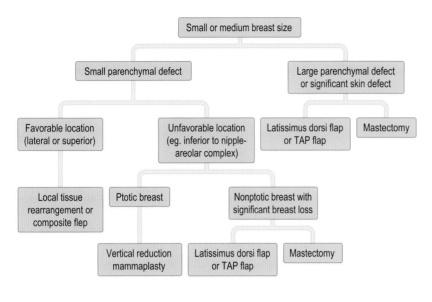

Figure 4.19 Treatment algorithm for immediate reconstruction after BCT versus mastectomy and reconstruction in order to optimize aesthetic outcome in small breasts. The smaller volume of tissue in the small breast limits local options for BCT compared to larger breasts. TAP (thoracodorsal artery perforator). Figure used with permission from Boughey, Oncoplastic Surgery for Breast Cancer, Chapter 13, in *Textbook of Surgical Oncology*, Poston GJ, Beauchamp R, Ruers T, eds, Taylor & Francis London and New York, 2008.

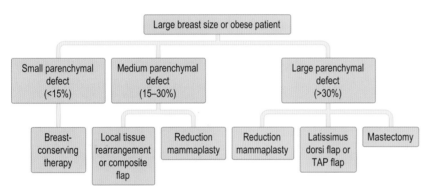

Figure 4.20 Treatment algorithm for immediate reconstruction after BCT versus mastectomy and reconstruction in order to optimize aesthetic outcome in large breasts. The larger breasts present a good option for BCT compared to smaller breasts. TAP (thoracodorsal artery perforator). Figure used with permission from Boughey, Oncoplastic Surgery for Breast Cancer, Chapter 13, in *Textbook of Surgical Oncology*, Poston GJ, Beauchamp R, Ruers T, eds, Taylor & Francis, London and New York, 2008.

References

1. NIH consensus conference. Treatment of early-stage breast cancer. JAMA 1991; 265(3):391–395.
2. Veronesi U, Luini A, Galimberti V, et al. Conservation approaches for the management of stage i/ii carcinoma of the breast: Milan cancer institute trials. World J Surg 1994; 18(1):70–75.
3. Arriagada R, Le MG, Rochard F, et al. Conservative treatment versus mastectomy in early breast cancer: patterns of failure with 15 years of follow-up data. Institut Gustave-Roussy Breast Cancer Group. J Clin Oncol 1996; 14(5):1558–1564.
4. Fisher B, Anderson S, Redmond CK, et al. Reanalysis and results after 12 years of follow-up in a randomized clinical trial comparing total mastectomy with lumpectomy with or without irradiation in the treatment of breast cancer. N Engl J Med 1995; 333(22):1456–1461.
5. Jacobson JA, Danforth DN, Cowan KH, et al. Ten-year results of a comparison of conservation with mastectomy in the treatment of stage i and ii breast cancer. N Engl J Med 1995; 332(14):907–911.

6. van Dongen JA, Voogd AC, Fentiman IS, et al. Long-term results of a randomized trial comparing breast-conserving therapy with mastectomy: European organization for research and treatment of cancer 10801 trial. J Natl Cancer Inst 2000; 92(14):1143–1150.
7. Blichert-Toft M, Rose C, Andersen JA, et al. Danish randomized trial comparing breast conservation therapy with mastectomy: six years of life-table analysis. Danish Breast Cancer Cooperative Group. J Natl Cancer Inst Monogr 1992; (11):19–25.
8. Clarke M, Collins R, Darby S, et al. Effects of radiotherapy and of differences in the extent of surgery for early breast cancer on local recurrence and 15-year survival: an overview of the randomized trials. Lancet 2005; 366(9503):2087–2106.
9. Petit JY, Rigaut L, Zekri A, et al. [Poor esthetic results after conservative treatment of breast cancer: technics of partial breast reconstruction]. Ann Chir Plast Esthet 1989; 34(2):103–108.
10. Olivotto IA, Rose MA, Osteen RT, et al. Late cosmetic outcome after conservative surgery and radiotherapy:

analysis of causes of cosmetic failure. Int J Radiat Oncol Biol Phys 1989; 17(4):747–753.
11. Abner AL, Recht A, Vicini FA, et al. Cosmetic results after surgery, chemotherapy, and radiation therapy for early breast cancer. Int J Radiat Oncol Biol Phys 1991; 21(2):331–338.
12. Bajaj AK, Kon PS, Oberg KC, et al. Aesthetic outcomes in patients undergoing breast conservation therapy for the treatment of localized breast cancer. Plast Reconstr Surg 2004; 114(6):1442–1449.
13. Rose MA, Olivotto I, Cady B, et al. Conservative surgery and radiation therapy for early breast cancer: long-term cosmetic results. Arch Surg 1989; 124(2):153–157.
14. Taylor ME, Perez CA, Halverson KJ, et al. Factors influencing cosmetic results after conservation therapy for breast cancer. Int J Radiat Oncol Biol Phys 1995; 31(4):753–764.
15. Choi JY, Alderman AK, Newman LA. Aesthetic and reconstruction considerations in oncologic breast surgery. J Am Coll Surg 2006; 2(6):943–952.

16. Clough KB, Cuminet J, Fitoussi A, Nos C, Mosseri V. Cosmetic sequelae after conservative treatment for breast cancer: classification and results of surgical correction. Ann Plast Surg 1998; 41(5):471–481.

17. Clough KB, Kroll SS, Audretsch W. An approach to the repair of partial mastectomy defects. Plast Reconstr Surg 1999; 104(2):409–420.

18. Clough KB, Lewis JS, Couturaud B, et al. Oncoplastic techniques allow extensive resections for breast-conserving therapy of breast carcinomas. Ann Surg 2003; 237(1):26–34.

19. D'Aniello C, Grimaldi L, Barbato A, et al. Cosmetic results in 242 patients treated by conservative surgery for breast cancer. Scand J Plast Reconstr Hand Surg 1999; 33:419–422.

20. Munhoz AM, Montag E, Arruda EG, et al. Critical analysis of reduction mammaplasty techniques in combination with conservative breast surgery for early breast cancer treatment. Plast Reconstr Surg 2006; 117(4):1091–1103.

21. Cocquyt VF, Blondeel PN, Depypere HT, et al. Better cosmetic results and comparable quality of life after skin-sparing mastectomy and immediate autologous breast reconstruction compared to breast conservative treatment. Br J Plast Surg 2003; 56:462–470.

22. Desch CE, Penberthy LT, Hillner BE, et al. A sociodemographic and economic comparison of breast reconstruction, mastectomy, and conservative surgery. Surgery 1999; 125(4):441–447.

23. Keating NL, Weeks JC, Borbas C, Guadagnoli E. Treatment of early stage breast cancer: do surgeons and patients agree regarding whether treatment alternatives were discussed? Breast Cancer Res Treat 2003; 79(2):225–231.

24. Nissen MJ, Swenson KK, Ritz LJ, et al. Quality of life after breast carcinoma surgery. a comparison of three surgical procedures. Cancer 2001; 91(7): 1238–1246.

25. Pusic A, Thompson TA, Kerrigan CL, et al. Surgical options for early-stage breast cancer: factors associated with patient choice and postoperative quality of life. Plast Reconstr Surg 1999; 104(5):1325–1333.

26. Moody AM, Mayles WP, Bliss JM, et al. The influence of breast size on late radiation effects and association with radiotherapy dose inhomogeneity. Radiother Oncol 1994; 33(2):106–112.

27. Olivotto IA, Rose MA, Osteen RT, et al. Late cosmetic outcome after conservative surgery and radiotherapy: analysis of causes of cosmetic failure. Int J Radiat Oncol Biol Phys 1989; 17(4):747–753.

28. Gray JR, McCormick B, Cox L, et al. Primary breast irradiation in large-breasted or heavy women: analysis of cosmetic outcome. Int J Radiat Oncol Biol Phys 1991; 21(2):347–354.

29. Montague ED, Paulus DD, Schell SR. Selection and follow-up of patients for conservation surgery and irradiation. Front Radiat Ther Oncol 1983; 17: 124–130.

30. Braw M, Erlandsson I, Ewers SB, Samuelsson L. Mammographic follow-up after breast conserving surgery and postoperative radiotherapy without boost irradiation for mammary carcinoma. Acta Radiol 1991; 32(5):398–402.

31. Berrino P, Campora E, Santi P. Postquadrantectomy breast deformities: classification and techniques of surgical correction. Plast Reconstr Surg 1987; 79(4):567–572.

32. Palit TK, Miltenburg DM, Brunicardi FC. Cost analysis of breast conservation surgery compared with modified radical mastectomy with and without reconstruction. Am J Surg 2000; 179:441–445.

33. Elkowitz A, Colen S, Slavin S, et al. Various methods of breast reconstruction after mastectomy: an economic comparison. Plast Reconstr Surg 1993; 92(1):77–83.

34. Khoo A, Kroll SS, Reece GP, et al. A comparison of resource costs of immediate and delayed breast reconstruction. Plast Reconstr Surg 1998; 101(4):964–970.

35. Lawrence GA. Cost-effective management of breast cancer. Am J Surg 2001; 182(4):435–436.

36. Spear SL, Burke JB, Forman D, et al. Experience with reduction mammaplasty following breast conservation surgery and radiation therapy. Plast Reconstr Surg 1998; 102(6):1913–1916.

37. Slavin SA, Love SM, Sadowsky NL. Reconstruction of the radiated partial mastectomy defect with autogenous tissues. Plast Reconstr Surg 1992; 90(5):854–865.

38. Smith ML, Evans GR, Gurlek A, et al. Reduction mammaplasty: its role in breast conservation surgery for early-stage breast cancer. Ann Plast Surg 1998; 41(3):234–239.

39. Stolier A, Allen R, Linares L. Breast conservation therapy with concomitant breast reduction in large-breasted women. Breast J 2003; 9(4):269–271.

40. Boughey JC, Peintinger F, Meric-Bernstam F, et al. Impact of preoperative versus postoperative chemotherapy on the extent and number of surgical procedures in patients treated in randomized clinical trials for breast cancer. Ann Surg 2006; 244(3):464–470.

41. Meric F, Mirza NQ, Vlastos G, et al. Positive surgical margins and ipsilateral breast tumor recurrence predict disease-specific survival after breast-conserving therapy. Cancer 2003; 97(4):926–933.

42. Barros A, Pinotti M, Ricci MD, et al. Immediate effects of intraoperative evaluation of surgical margins over the treatment of early infiltrating breast carcinoma. Tumori 2003; 89(1):42–45.

43. Chagpar A, Yen T, Sahin A, et al. Intraoperative margin assessment reduces reexcision rates in patients with ductal carcinoma in situ treated with breast-conserving surgery. Am J Surg 2003; 186(4):371–377.

44. Bold RJ, Kroll SS, Baldwin BJ, Ross MI, Singletary SE. Local rotational flaps for breast conservation therapy as an alternative to mastectomy. Ann Surg Oncol 1997; 4(7):540–544.

45. Bruhlmann Y, Tschopp H. Breast reduction improves symptoms of macromastia and has a long-lasting effect. Ann Plast Surg 1998; 41(3): 240–245.

46. Boice JD Jr, Persson I, Brinton LA, et al. Breast cancer following breast reduction surgery in Sweden. Plast Reconstr Surg 2000; 106(4):755–762.

47. Brown MH, Weinberg M, Chong N, et al. A cohort study of breast cancer risk in breast reduction patients. Plast Reconstr Surg 1999; 103(6): 1674–1681.

48. Jansen DA, Murphy M, Kind GM, et al. Breast cancer in reduction mammoplasty: case reports and a survey of plastic surgeons. Plast Reconstr Surg 1998; 101(2):361–364.

49. Handel N, Lewinsky B, Waisman JR. Reduction mammaplasty following radiation therapy for breast cancer. Plast Reconstr Surg 1992; 89(5): 953–955.

50. Losken A, Elwood ET, Styblo TM, et al. The role of reduction mammaplasty in reconstructing partial mastectomy defects. Plast Reconstr Surg 2002; 109(3):968–975; discussion 76–77.

51. Maxwell GP. Iginio tansini and the origin of the latissimus dorsi musculocutaneous flap. Plast Reconstr Surg 1980; 65(5):686–692.

52. Kronowitz SJ, Feledy JA, Hunt KK, et al. Determining the optimal approach to breast reconstruction after partial mastectomy. Plast Reconstr Surg 2006; 117(1):1–11.

53. Tobin GR, Schusterman M, Peterson GH, et al. The intramuscular neurovascular anatomy of the latissimus dorsi muscle: the basis for splitting the flap. Plast Reconstr Surg 1981; 67(5):637–641.

54. Angrigiani C, Grilli D, Siebert J. Latissimus dorsi musculocutaneous flap without muscle. Plast Reconstr Surg 1995; 96(7):1608–1614.

55. Hamdi M, Van Landuyt K, Monstrey S, et al. Pedicled perforator flaps in breast reconstruction: a new concept. Br J Plast Surg 2004; 57(6):531–539.

56. Thomas PR, Ford HT, Gazet JC. Use of silicone implants after wide local excision of the breast. Br J Surg 1993; 80(7):868–870.

57. Coleman SR, Saboeiro AP. Fat grafting to the breast revisited: safety and efficacy. Plast Reconstr Surg 2007; 119(3):775–785.

58. Rigotte G, Marchi A, Galie M, et al. Plast Reconstr Surg 2007; 119(5):1409–1422.

45

CHAPTER 5

Oncoplastic Breast Conservation Surgery

Melvin J Silverstein

Introduction

Oncoplastic breast conservation surgery combines oncologic principles with plastic surgical techniques. But it is much more than a combination of two disciplines – it is a philosophy that requires vision, passion, a knowledge of anatomy, and an appreciation and understanding of aesthetics, symmetry and breast function. The oncoplastic surgeon must be constantly thinking 'How can I remove this cancer with large margins of normal tissue while at the same time making the patient look as good or better than she looks now?' (**Box 5.1**).

The ultimate oncoplastic achievement would be to convert what would normally be an oncologic and/or cosmetic failure using standard techniques into both an oncologic and cosmetic success. Avoiding mastectomy when it seems inevitable and ending with an excellent cosmetic result is one way to achieve that goal. The following case demonstrates just such a scenario.

A 58-year-old female presented with recurrent ductal carcinoma in situ (DCIS) in the left lower inner quadrant of the breast. A previous excision had been performed 2 years earlier obtaining a minimal margin of clearance. The left breast was severely deformed following this procedure (**Fig. 5.1**). Following the local recurrence, she was told by multiple surgeons that mastectomy was the only option. After re-evaluation, including digital mammography, ultrasound, and magnetic resonance imaging (MRI), it was determined that the only disease present was at the edge of the previous excision. A left wire-directed segmental resection using a reduction incision with a contralateral (right) reduction was performed (**Figs 5.2–5.5**). This procedure excised the residual DCIS with a margin of excision that exceeded 10 mm in all directions. The cosmetic appearance was much improved and was persistent 4 years later (**Fig. 5.6**).

The history of oncoplastic breast conservation surgery in the United States

There is little written about the origins of oncoplastic breast conservation surgery in the United States. We began developing oncoplastic techniques in the early 1980s by accident.

The first free-standing Breast Center in the United States was founded in Van Nuys, California, in 1979.[1,2] Our group consisted of plastic surgeons, oncologic surgeons, medical oncologists, radiologists, radiation oncologists, and a psychiatrist. In the early years, due to staffing issues it was not uncommon for an oncologic surgeon to assist a plastic surgeon with a reduction and for a plastic surgeon to assist an oncologic surgeon with a mastectomy or

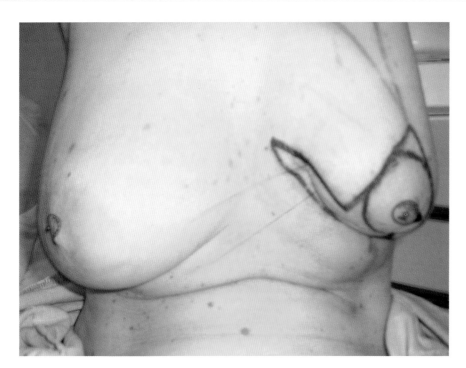

Figure 5.1 A 58-year-old white female presented with recurrent DCIS in the left lower inner quadrant. She had been excised twice, 2 years earlier. Minimal clear margins were achieved but the left breast was severely deformed. She was advised to have a left mastectomy by multiple surgeons.

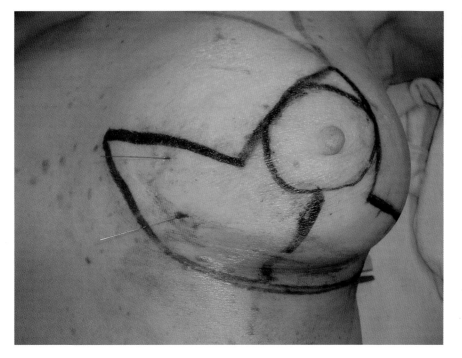

Figure 5.2 The plan for excision using a reduction pattern. Two wires are in place, bracketing the calcifications marking the recurrence.

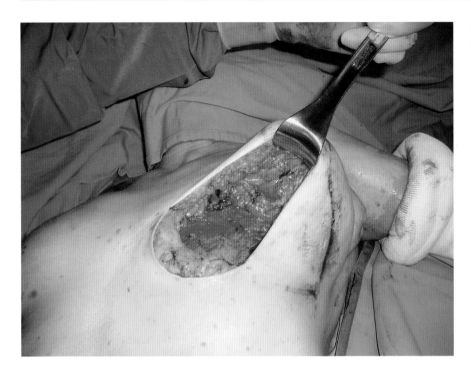

Figure 5.3 The lower inner quadrant has been excised.

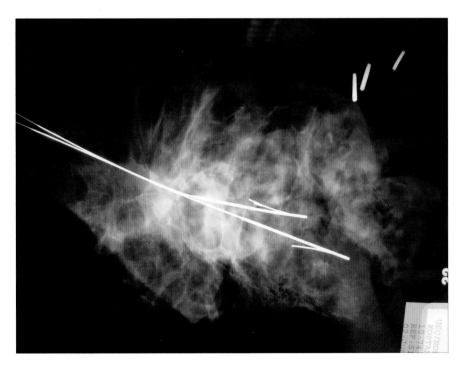

Figure 5.4 Specimen radiograph shows the excised calcifications with widely clear margins radiographically.

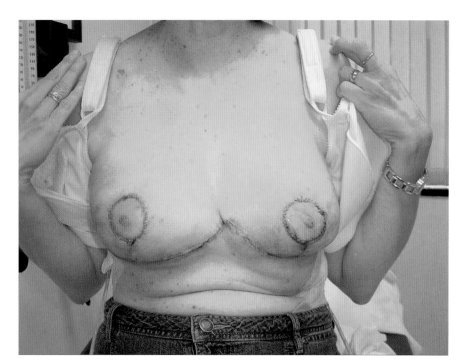

Figure 5.5 The patient is 5 days postoperative with drains in place.

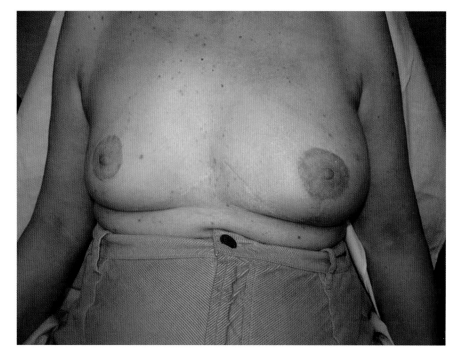

Figure 5.6 The patient is 4 years postoperative without recurrence. The cosmetic result has been maintained.

Box 5.1

The goals of oncoplastic breast conservation surgery include:

1. Complete removal of the lesion
2. Clear margins – the larger the better
3. Good to excellent cosmetic result
4. Going to the operating room one time to perform the definitive procedure

axillary dissection. Because of this, both disciplines (plastic and oncologic surgery) became quite familiar with what the other discipline could accomplish.

Our first true oncoplastic case occurred in 1982. A young pregnant woman was referred with a biopsy-proven giant fibroadenoma of pregnancy (**Fig. 5.7**). We waited until she delivered her baby and then a few weeks later a team of one oncologic and one plastic surgeon removed the benign tumor using a reduction approach and simultaneously reduced the opposite side (**Fig. 5.8**). Owing to the large size of the tumor (about 20 cm), the nipples ended up a bit too high, but overall it was an outstanding oncoplastic result (**Fig. 5.9**).

Shortly thereafter, one of our plastic surgeons did a reduction by removing a large segment of superior breast tissue in an older woman who did not want a standard reduction. When asked what he called this strange incision, he answered 'Batwing … because it looks like the Batman symbol.' At the same time, we were learning more about the importance of widely clear margins, something that had not been appreciated prior to the mid 1980s. We quickly adopted the 'batwing' for women with breast cancer in the upper half of a larger breast that could benefit from lifting of the nipple–areola complex (NAC). The rest, as they say, is history. We rapidly added more

and varied excisions to our 'oncoplastic' armamentarium, many of which will be illustrated below.

Oncoplastic resection

When treating a patient with biopsy-proven breast cancer, the non-oncoplastic approach would be to make a small cosmetically placed curvilinear incision over the area to be removed (**Fig. 5.10**). This would typically include no skin and a relatively small piece of breast tissue. The definition of a clear margin was based on non-transection of the tumor. Complete and sequential tissue processing is not usually performed and postoperative radiation therapy is the usual protocol.

But the trend is changing. During the last 25 years, my colleagues and I have developed a comprehensive multidisciplinary oncoplastic approach for the excision of breast cancer.[3–5] It requires surgical coordination with a pathologist, a radiologist and, often, a plastic surgeon. Oncoplastic surgery combines sound surgical oncologic principles with plastic surgical techniques. Coordination of the two surgical disciplines may help to avoid poor cosmetic results after wide excision and may increase the number of women who can be treated with breast-conserving surgery by allowing larger breast excisions with more acceptable cosmetic results. These techniques are applicable to patients with both noninvasive (DCIS) and invasive breast cancer.

Oncoplastic resection is a therapeutic procedure, not a breast biopsy. It is performed on patients with a proven diagnosis of breast cancer. This approach was strongly supported by the 2005 Consensus Conference on Image-Detected Breast Cancer.[6] An important goal in caring for a woman with breast cancer is to go to the operating room a single time and to perform a definitive procedure

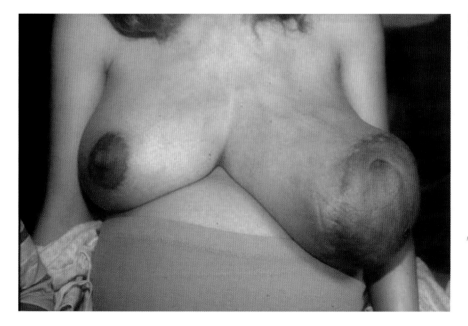

Figure 5.7 A 27-year-old pregnant patient with a biopsy-proven giant fibroadenoma of pregnancy.

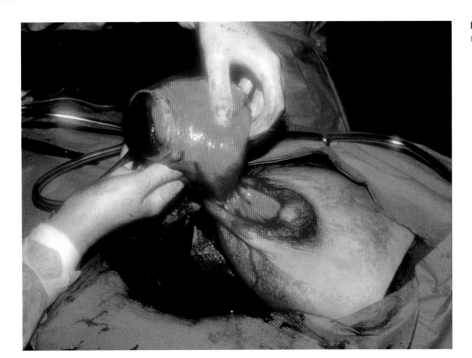

Figure 5.8 The tumor was excised and measures 20 cm.

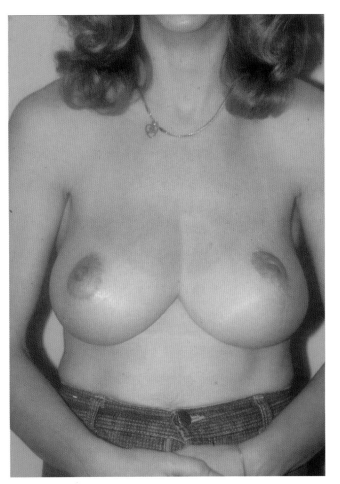

Figure 5.9 Redundant skin was excised using a reduction pattern and the contralateral breast reduced. The patient is pictured here 7 years postoperative.

that does not require re-operation. Whenever possible, the initial breast biopsy should be made using a minimally invasive percutaneous technique.[6] This usually provides ample tissue for diagnosis.

When excising breast cancer, the surgeon faces two opposing goals: clear margins versus an acceptable cosmetic result. From an oncologic point of view, the largest specimen possible should be removed in an attempt to achieve the widest possible margins. From a cosmetic point of view, a much smaller amount of tissue should be removed in order to achieve the best possible cosmetic result. The surgeon must tread a fine line as he or she tries to satisfy two masters. The first attempt to remove a cancerous lesion is critical. The first excision offers the best chance to remove the entire lesion in one piece, evaluate its extent and margin status, and to achieve the best possible cosmetic result.

Currently, as many as 40–50% of new breast cancer cases are discovered by modern state-of-the-art imaging (mostly mammography) and, intraoperatively, are grossly both non-palpable and non-visualizable. Under these circumstances, the surgeon essentially operates blindly. Multiple hooked wires can help define the extent of the lesion radiographically. Using bracketing wires, the surgeon should make an attempt to excise the entire lesion within a single piece of tissue. This often will include overlying skin as well as pectoral fascia (**Figs 5.11** and **5.12**). The tissue should be precisely oriented for the pathologist.

If the specimen is removed in multiple pieces rather than a single piece, there is little likelihood of evaluating margins and size accurately. **Figure 5.13** shows an excision

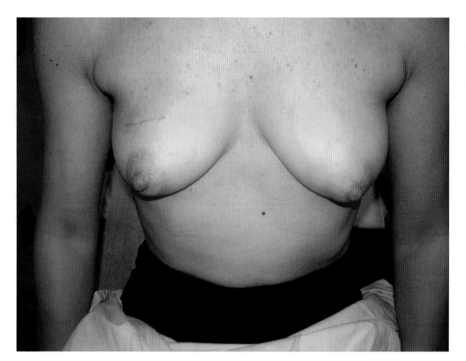

Figure 5.10 A patient with biopsy-proven breast cancer. The cancer has been excised through a small cosmetically placed curvilinear incision over the lesion. No skin has been removed. Until now, this has been the standard way of excising breast cancer.

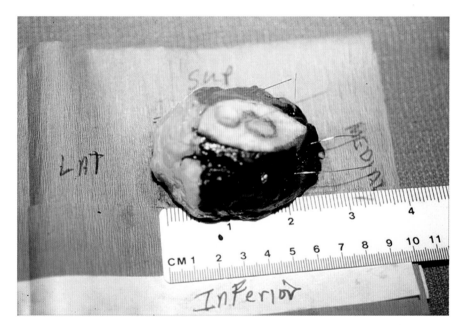

Figure 5.11 An excised, color-coded specimen (from skin to fascia) with guide wires in place.

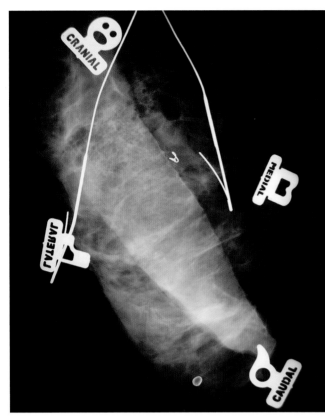

Figure 5.12 Intraoperative specimen radiography showing skin, bracketing wires, clip marking the biopsy cavity, and the specimen oriented using Margin Map (Beekley, Inc, Bristol, CT).

specimen with four additional pieces that allegedly represent the new margins. The additional pieces are too small and do not reflect the true margins of the original specimen. If one makes a judgment on margin clearance based on these small additional pieces, that judgment might very well be incorrect.

Oncoplastic steps

There are several important steps to a proper oncoplastic operation.

1. Preoperative planning (includes surgeon and radiologist) and should include:
   (a) mammography (preferably digital);
   (b) breast ultrasound (at a minimum, the involved quadrant but preferably both breasts);
   (c) axillary ultrasound and needle biopsy, if indicated;
   (d) breast MRI;
   (e) an evaluation of the size of the cancer versus the size of the breast;
   (f) detailed family history and genetic counseling, if appropriate;
   (g) integration of patient wishes.
2. Excision of lesion in one piece (often includes skin, breast segment and pectoral fascia).
3. Reshape the breast.
4. Symmetry.

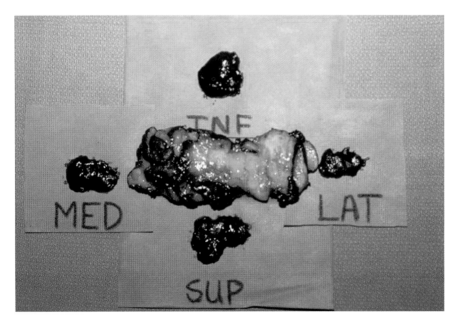

Figure 5.13 An excision specimen with four additional pieces of tissue that allegedly represent the new margins. The additional pieces are too small and do not reflect the true margins of the original specimen. If one makes a judgment on margin clearance based on these small additional pieces, that judgment might very well be wrong.

Preoperative planning requires discussion between the oncoplastic surgeon and the radiologist. All of the preoperative tests must be evaluated and integrated along with information about the pathologic subtype of the lesion. Is it an invasive lobular cancer that might be larger than expected? Is there a significant DCIS component? Does this patient want symmetry? If yes, should it be done during the same operative procedure or as a delayed procedure? And so on.

Oncoplastic excisions

There are a wide range of oncoplastic incisions. These include:

1. Upper pole:
   (a) crescent;
   (b) batwing;
   (c) hemi-batwing;
2. Lower pole:
   (a) triangle;
   (b) trapezoid;
   (c) reduction;
   (d) inframammary (hidden scar) (does not remove skin);
3. Any segment of the breast:
   (a) radial – ellipse (most versatile);
   (b) circumareola with advancement flap (does not remove skin);
   (c) donut mastopexy.

Some of these excisions are illustrated below, using selected cases.

Radial ellipse

Figure 5.14 shows the preoperative markings for a patient with a lesion in the 9:00 position of the right breast. Three wheals of isosulfan blue dye have been injected intradermally for sentinel node localization. (Do not use intradermal injections unless skin is going to be removed. It will tattoo the skin.) The entire lateral segment down to and including the pectoralis major fascia was removed and the surrounding tissue undermined (**Fig. 5.15**). A sentinel node biopsy was performed. The remaining tissue was then advanced with deep sutures and the breast remodeled (**Fig. 5.16**). **Figures 5.17–5.20** show the cosmetic results of radial elliptical excisions.

Following segmental resections, all women will have drains inserted that will remain for 24–48 hours (Fig. 5.19). All incisions are closed in a layered fashion. The cosmetic result should be constantly monitored and reappraised during wound closure. It is prudent to elevate the head of the operating table to re-evaluate the cosmetic result and symmetry.

A radial segmental resection may alter the size and shape of the breast but good cosmetic results are usually achieved (Figs 5.17–5.20). A radial excision generally will not displace the NAC even though overlying skin is removed. If it does, the nipple can be re-centralized by excising a crescent-shaped piece of skin (see crescent excision below).

In contrast to the old axiom 'the seroma is your friend', when doing oncoplastic breast surgery the exact opposite is true. It is best if the wound heals with as little seroma and blood as possible. Regardless of how the wound is

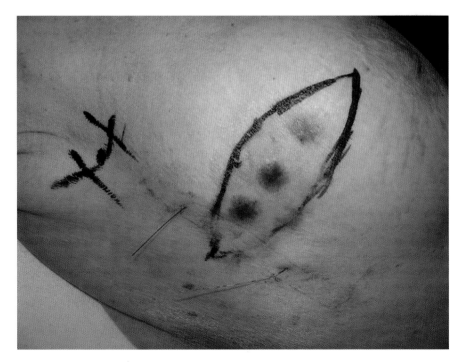

Figure 5.14 Preoperative markings for a patient with a lesion in the 9:00 position of the right breast. Three wheals of isosulfan blue dye have been injected intradermally for sentinel node localization. The sentinel node incision has been marked.

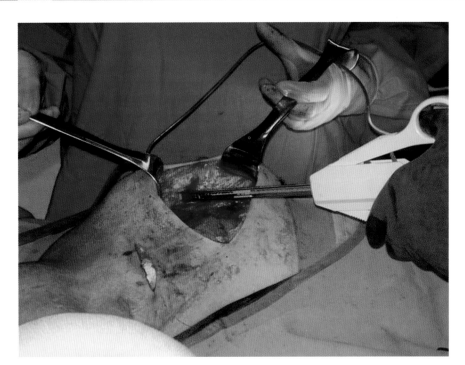

Figure 5.15 The entire lateral segment down to and including the pectoralis major fascia has been removed and the surrounding tissue undermined. Clips are used to mark the superior, inferior, medial, lateral and deep margins of the excision. A sentinel node biopsy has been performed.

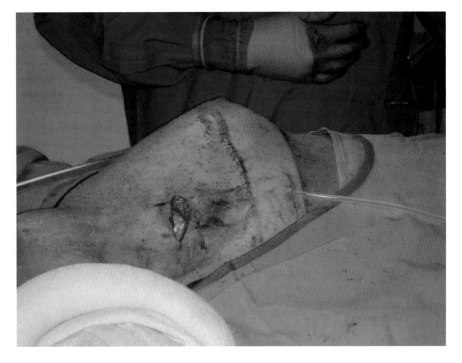

Figure 5.16 The remaining tissue has been advanced with deep sutures and the breast remodeled. The skin has been clipped together prior to suturing and the breast has been drained through a small incision in the inframammary sulcus.

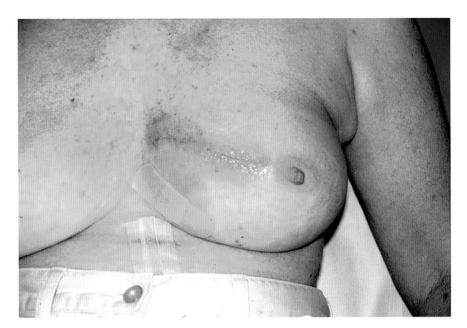

Figure 5.17 The result of a radial ellipse in the upper inner quadrant of the left breast. The skin has been closed with a subcuticular suture and Dermabond (Ethicon, Inc., Cincinnati, OH). The patient is 4 days postoperative.

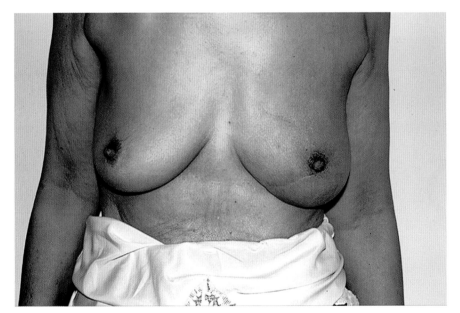

Figure 5.18 The result of a radial ellipse in the lower inner quadrant of the left breast. The patient is 2 years postoperative.

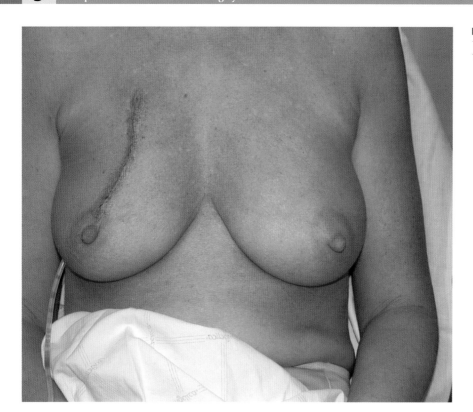

Figure 5.19 The result of a radial ellipse in the 12:00 position of the right breast. The patient is 1 day postoperative.

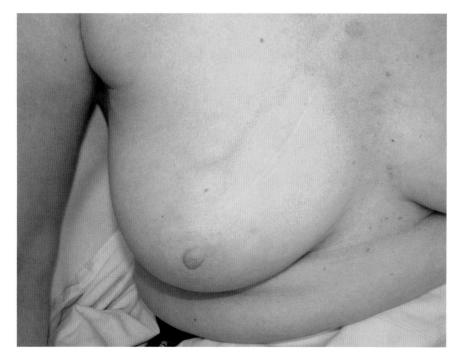

Figure 5.20 The result of a radial ellipse in the upper inner quadrant of the right breast. The patient is 2 years postoperative.

closed, there will always be a small amount of fluid in the biopsy cavity, but this should be minimized.

Segmentectomy using a variety of reduction mammoplasty excisions

In a fully counseled woman with a larger breast, who might benefit from a reduction mammoplasty or a mastopexy, and whose breast cancer is in the right position (generally the lower half of the breast), a variety of creative reduction/mastopexy excisions can be designed that allow for complete removal of the lesion.

For lesions in the lower hemisphere of the breast a standard reduction incision can be used.[7] This allows access to lesions from 3:00 to 9:00, going clockwise. Large amounts of breast tissue can be removed with excellent cosmetic results and generally widely clear margins.

A 65-year-old woman presented with needle biopsy proven DCIS in the right breast. The DCIS was central with a bloody nipple discharge. It was elected to do a wide local excision, including the NAC, using two guide wires and a reduction pattern (**Fig. 5.21**). **Figures 5.22–5.25** show the details of the procedure and early results.

Triangle

The triangle excision removes a triangle-shaped piece of tissue from the lower hemisphere of the breast (generally from the 5:00, 6:00 or 7:00 position). It does not elevate the NAC. **Figure 5.26** shows a 48-year-old patient with an invasive lesion in the 5:30 position on the left breast. It was removed through a curvilinear incision but the superior margin was positive. An MRI revealed residual disease

in the left breast extending toward the nipple. **Figures 5.27** and **5.28** show the details of the procedure and final result.

Inframammary approach (hidden scar)

The inframammary approach places the incision in the inframammary sulcus and is generally invisible with the patient in the upright position. This incision is an excellent choice for lesions in the posterior inferior portion of the breast. It does not remove any skin. **Figures 5.29–5.35** detail a 51-year-old patient with a 1 cm lesion in the posterior lateral breast.

Crescent, batwing and hemi-batwing

For lesions in the upper hemisphere (8 o'clock to 4 o'clock, going clockwise), crescent, batwing or hemi-batwing excisions can be used. These incisions allow the lesion to be generously removed (specimens are often 200 g or more) while allowing recontouring of the breast in a desirable fashion. All will elevate the position of the NAC. **Figures 5.36** and **5.37** show a woman whose lesion in the 12 o'clock position of the left breast was excised using a crescent mastopexy incision. **Figure 5.38** shows a patient with large breasts with a cancer in the 12:00 position of the left breast. She could have benefited from bilateral batwing excisions but she refused to have anything done on the right. Because we did not want to create too much asymmetry, we raised the left NAC only 5 cm (**Fig. 5.39**).

Figures 5.40 and **5.41** show a patient with bilateral DCIS who was excised using bilateral hemi-batwing

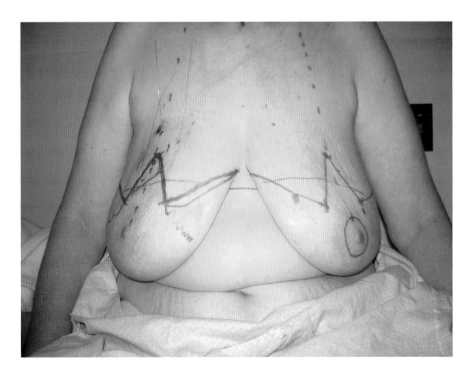

Figure 5.21 A 65-year-old woman presented with needle biopsy proven DCIS in the right breast. The DCIS was central with a bloody nipple discharge. It was elected to do a wide local excision, including the NAC, using two guide wires and a reduction pattern.

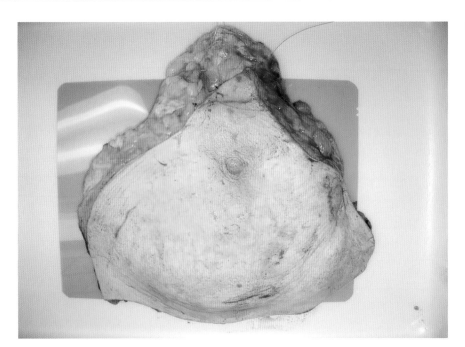

Figure 5.22 The excised lower central segment, including the NAC, of the right breast.

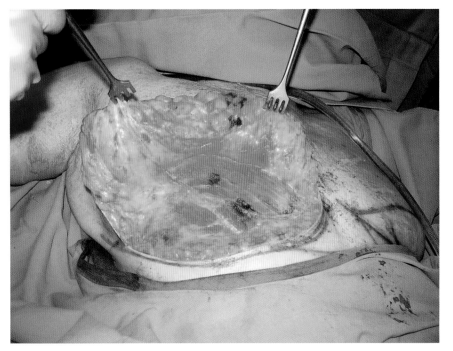

Figure 5.23 The lower central segment of the right breast has been removed, the incisions along the inframammary sulcus have been lengthened, and the remaining breast has been undermined from the chest wall.

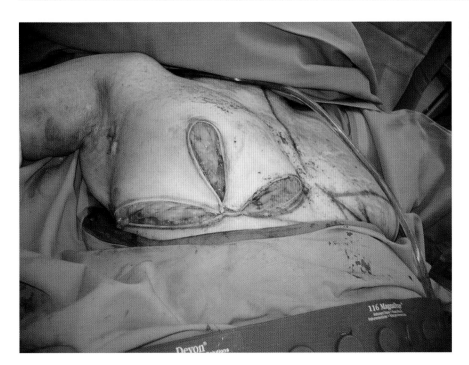

Figure 5.24 The remaining tissue has been re-approximated and will be closed with deep sutures. A sentinel node biopsy has been done through a separate incision but it could have been done through the reduction incision by extending the undermining to the lower axilla.

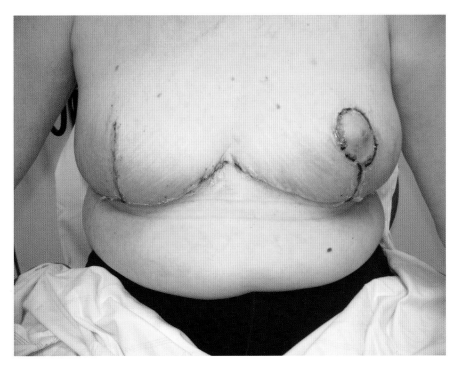

Figure 5.25 The patient is 2 weeks postoperative. The lower central segment of the right breast, including the NAC, has been removed through a reduction incision and the left breast has been reduced to match the right. The right NAC will be created about 3 months postoperatively.

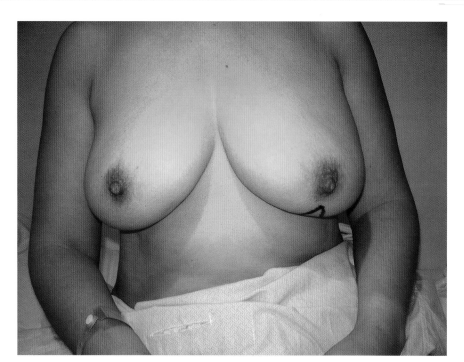

Figure 5.26 A 48-year-old patient with an invasive lesion in the 5:30 position of the left breast.

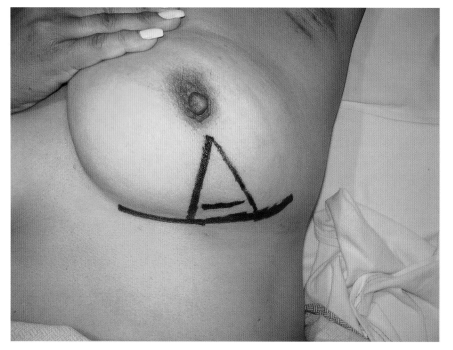

Figure 5.27 The lesion was removed through a curvilinear incision in the 5:30 position (marked in black ink) but the superior margin was positive. An MRI revealed residual disease in the left breast extending toward the nipple. A triangle-shaped excision has been drawn on the breast to allow re-excision of the entire segment from inframammary sulcus to the nipple.

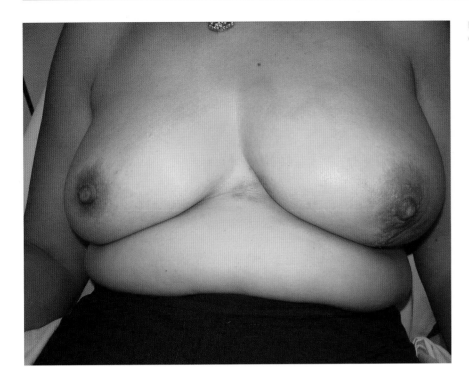

Figure 5.28 The patient is 1 week post triangle excision in the left breast.

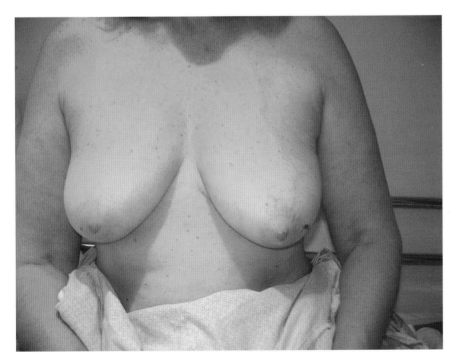

Figure 5.29 A 51-year-old patient with a 1 cm lesion in the posterior lateral left breast.

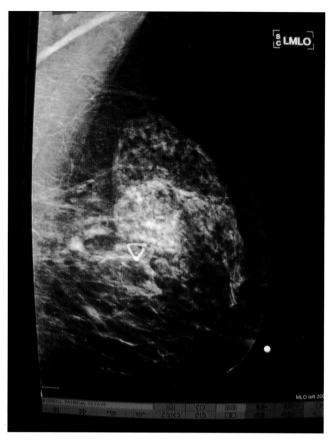

Figure 5.30 Mediolateral mammogram shows the lesion about nipple high and posterior in the left breast. Triangle marks the lesion.

excisions. Widely clear margins were obtained on both sides. The hemi-batwing is a combination of a radial ellipse and a crescent excision. It is designed to raise the NAC while excising a radial segment of the breast.

The contralateral breast

When symmetry is desired, the contralateral breast will generally need to be adjusted. This can be done during the same operative procedure as the initial cancer or as a delayed procedure. The advantage of doing both sides simultaneously is obvious: a single operative procedure. The disadvantage is that the final pathology and, in particular, the margin status are unknown before altering the appearance of the opposite breast. However, if the patient decides that she is willing to accept the risks of close or positive margins (that might require reoperation) and would prefer a single operation, the contralateral side can be adjusted at the same operation.

If permanent microscopic sections reveal involved margins and the residual breast is amenable to re-excision, the inflammatory response and induration should be allowed to subside if the re-excision is for DCIS. If the re-excision is for invasive cancer, it can be done immediately or after the completion of chemotherapy (if indicated) but prior to radiation therapy. The cosmetic results from re-excision are often better after a sufficient period of wound healing and scar resolution.

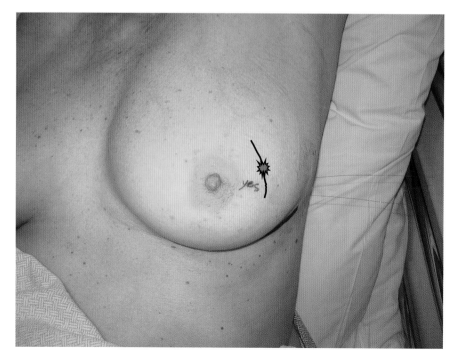

Figure 5.31 Shows the patient ready for surgery. Two guide wires are in place marking the lesion. Ultrasound has been used intraoperatively to map out the exact position of the lesion (pink stellate cartoon) and a curvilinear black line has been drawn in natural skin lines to show how most surgeons would approach this lesion.

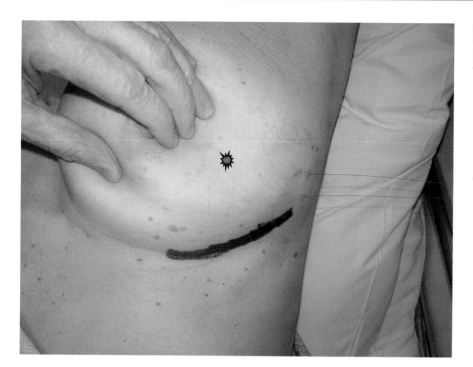

Figure 5.32 Rather than a curvilinear incision over the lesion, the approach will be using an inframammary incision with ultrasound assistance throughout the procedure.

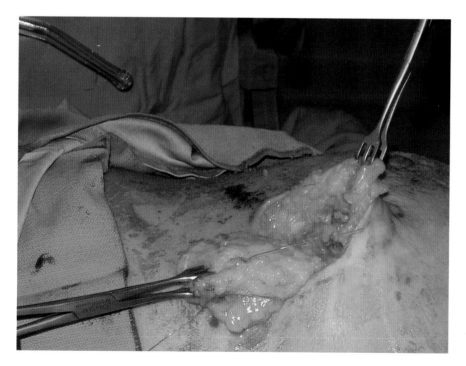

Figure 5.33 The posterior portion of the breast is being excised with both guide wires in place.

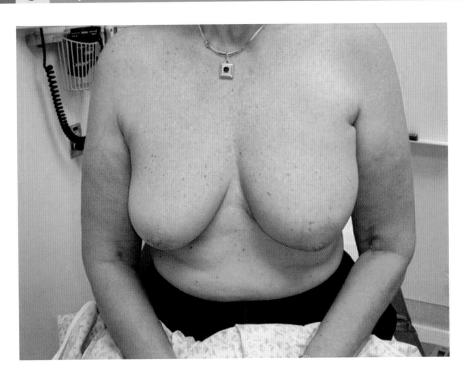

Figure 5.34 The patient is 18 months post inframammary excision followed by radiation therapy. The incision is invisible unless the breast is pulled superiorly.

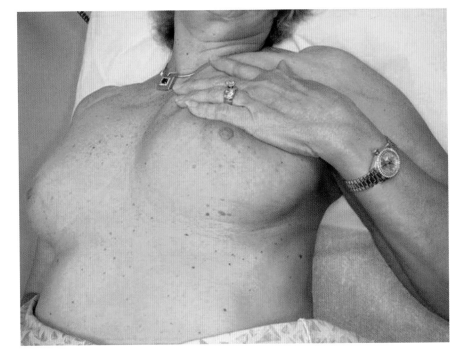

Figure 5.35 The breast has been pulled superiorly and the incision is barely visible as a fine white line.

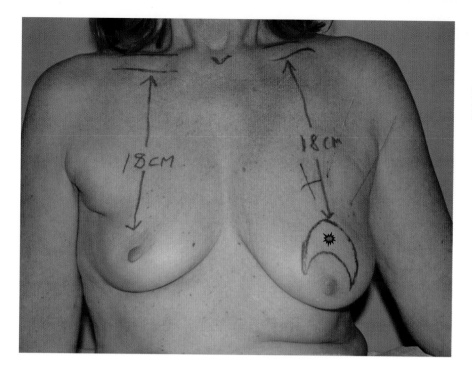

Figure 5.36 A 52-year-old patient treated 8 years previously for carcinoma of the right breast. She now presents with a mirror image lesion in the left breast (pink cartoon). Measurements have been made and it was decided to elevate the left nipple to 18 cm below the midpoint of the clavicle. The left breast lesion is marked by two bracketing wires.

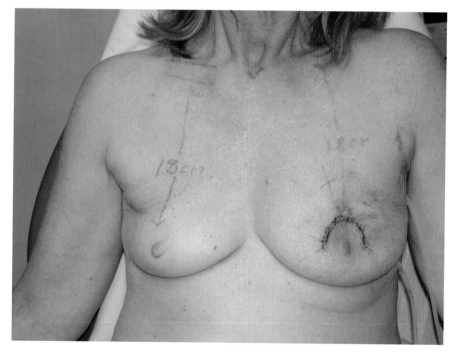

Figure 5.37 The patient is 1 day postoperative. Excellent symmetry has been achieved and the cancer has been removed with widely clear margins.

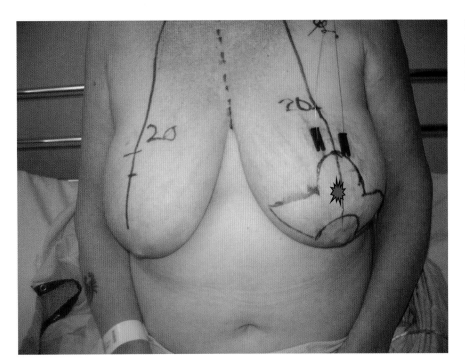

Figure 5.38 A patient with large breasts with a cancer in the 12:00 position of the left breast (pink cartoon). The lesion is marked by two bracketing wires. She could have benefited from bilateral batwing excisions but she refused to have anything done on the right.

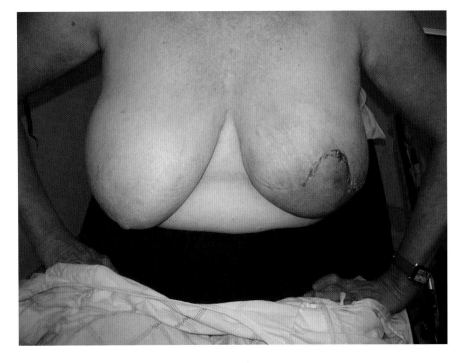

Figure 5.39 Because we did not want to create too much asymmetry, we raised the left NAC only 5 cm. She is 10 days postoperative in this picture.

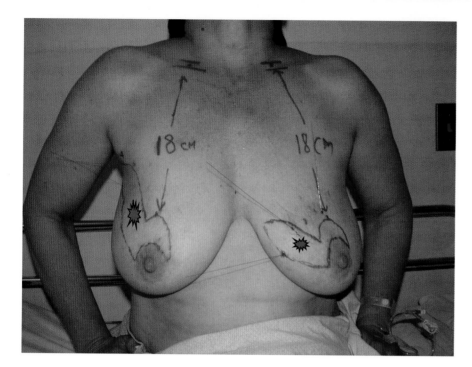

Figure 5.40 A 55-year-old patient with bilateral DCIS (the right upper outer quadrant and the left upper inner quadrant. Both lesions are marked by pink cartoons. Two bracketing wires are in place on the right and three on the left.)

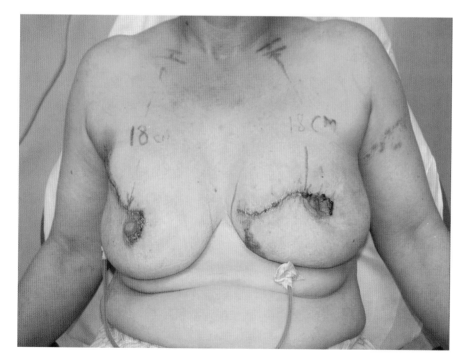

Figure 5.41 The patient is 1 day postoperative. The NACs have been raised to 18 cm below the mid-portion of the clavicles. Drains are in place on both sides and will be removed. Final pathology revealed excellent margins on both sides.

Summary

Oncoplastic surgery combines sound surgical oncologic principles with plastic surgical techniques. Coordination of the two surgical disciplines may help to avoid poor cosmetic results after wide excision and may increase the number of women who can be treated with breast-conserving surgery by allowing larger breast excisions with more acceptable cosmetic results. Oncoplastic surgery requires cooperation and coordination of surgical oncology, radiology, and pathology. Oncoplastic resection is a therapeutic procedure, not a breast biopsy, and is performed on patients with a proven diagnosis of breast cancer.

References

1. Silverstein MJ. The Van Nuys Breast Center: the first free-standing multidisciplinary breast center. Surg Oncol Clin North Am 2000; 9(2): 159–175.
2. Silverstein MJ, Handel N, Hoffman R, et al. The breast center: a multidisciplinary model. In: Paterson AHG, ed. Fundamental problems in breast cancer. Martinus Nijhoff: Boston, MA; 1987:47–58.
3. Silverstein MJ, Larsen L, Soni R, et al. Breast biopsy and oncoplastic surgery for the patient with ductal carcinoma in situ: surgical, pathologic and radiologic issues. In: Silverstein MJ, Recht A, Lagios M, eds. Ductal carcinoma in situ of the breast. Lippincott, Williams & Wilkins: Philadelphia; 2002:185–206.
4. Anderson B, Masetti R, Silverstein M. Oncoplastic approaches to partial mastectomy: an overview of volume displacement techniques. Lancet Oncol 2005; 6:145–157.
5. Silverstein MJ. An argument against routine use of radiotherapy for ductal carcinoma in situ. Oncology 2003; 17(11):1511–1546.
6. Silverstein M, Lagios M, Recht A, et al. Image-detected breast cancer: state of the art diagnosis and treatment. J Am Coll Surg 2005; 201:586–597.
7. Clough K, Lewis J, Couturaud B, et al. Oncoplastic techniques allow extensive resections for breast conserving therapy of breast carcinomas. Ann Surg 2003; 237:26–34.

CHAPTER 6

Reduction Mammaplasty and Oncoplastic Surgery

Albert Losken

Introduction

There has been a significant increase in the popularity of mammaplasty techniques being used for the reconstruction of partial mastectomy defects prior to breast irradiation for women with early-stage breast cancer. This has been fueled in part by the ever-expanding indications for breast conservation therapy (BCT), and the desire to improve outcomes from an oncologic standpoint as well as a cosmetic one. Although breast-sparing surgery has demonstrated equivalent survival rates,[1,2] poor cosmetic results are not uncommon in certain patients. One such group of patients are those with large or ptotic breasts. Macromastia was initially felt to be a relative contraindication to BCT with poor cosmetic results and less effective radiation therapy.[3] Radiation-induced fibrosis is felt to be greater in women with larger breasts, given the dosing inhomogeneity.[4,5] Late-radiation fibrosis has been demonstrated 36% of the time in patients with larger breasts, compared to 3.6% for smaller breasts.[5] Higher doses of radiation therapy are often necessary in women with larger breasts, contributing to morbidity and adversely affecting the appearance. The cosmetic results following BCT in women with large breasts are also reduced. Clarke has shown excellent results in 100% of women with A-cup breasts following BCT, compared to 50% in women with D-cup breasts.[6] On the other hand, women with macromastia and large pendulous breasts are often overweight, and total breast reconstruction is more challenging, being associated with higher complication rates and less favorable cosmetic outcomes. The addition of reduction mammaplasty techniques was therefore welcomed by the patient, the ablative surgeon and the reconstructive surgeon. It allows women with macromastia to be candidates for breast conservation without having to accept significant deformities, allows the ablative surgeon to remove a generous amount without having to worry about a residual deformity, and it makes breast reconstruction more predictable in an otherwise difficult patient population. In addition to the many potential benefits of combining these two techniques, the disadvantages in well-selected patients are minimal. Oncoplastic reduction techniques initially became popular in Europe for reconstructing quadrantectomy defects in the lower pole.[7] In the United States, their popularity likely evolved out of frustration in the management of breast cancer patients with macromastia, however, and is now one of the most common methods used for reconstructing partial mastectomy defects at the time of resection.[8-10] As long as we continue to demonstrate high levels of patient safety and patient satisfaction, the oncoplastic reduction techniques will likely become even more popular in the future.

Indications

The indications for using oncoplastic reduction techniques are numerous. In addition to the cosmetic and oncologic reasons, the quality-of-life benefits to breast reduction surgery for women with macromastia have already been demonstrated. The two main reasons to reconstruct partial mastectomy defects are: (1) to increase the indications for BCT, making breast conservation practical in patients who otherwise might require a mastectomy; and (2) to minimize the potential for a poor aesthetic result (**Table 6.1**). The decision is usually based on tumor characteristics (size and location) and breast characteristics (size and shape).

Women with large pendulous breasts who are felt by the surgeon to be poor candidates for BCT alone benefit from the oncoplastic reduction techniques, minimizing the potential for a poor cosmetic result and allowing them to be candidates for breast conservation (**Fig. 6.1**). The ideal patient is one whose tumor can be widely excised within the reduction specimen, and for whom a smaller breast is viewed as a positive outcome. Older women with macromastia are well suited for this approach compared to mastectomy and reconstruction (**Fig. 6.2**). Another indication for the oncoplastic reduction technique is when the surgeon anticipates a large defect, or is concerned about being able to achieve clear margins in women with moderate to large breasts. The potential for an unfavorable result exists in this situation regardless of breast size or tumor location. Other indications are patient driven, in those women who desire breast conservation, or who desire smaller breasts due to their limitations caused by symptomatic macromastia. As we become more comfortable with these techniques, the indications will become more liberal. Essentially anyone with large breasts amenable to breast conservation is a candidate for this procedure. However, the importance of stringent patient selection criteria cannot be overstated, and is required to ensure maximal cosmetic outcomes as well as oncological safety.

Table 6.1 Indications for reconstruction of partial mastectomy defects

Cosmetic reasons	Oncologic reasons
High tumor to breast ratio (>20%)	Concern about clear margins
Tumor location: central, inferior, medial	Wide excision required
Macromastia	Poor candidate for mastectomy and reconstruction (i.e., age, breast size)
Large tumor	Patient desires BCT
Patient desires smaller breasts	More effective radiation therapy
Significant ptosis, or breast asymmetry	Quality-of-life benefits

Contraindications include patients who are not good candidates for breast conservation, a history of prior irradiation or situations when there is insufficient residual breast tissue following resection to allow reshaping. Similar selection criteria are used when deciding on elective breast reduction procedures and need to be taken into consideration. Patients with multiple medical comorbidities or active smokers are not ideal candidates for additional elective surgery, and the risks will often outweigh the benefits in these situations.

Patient selection and margin status

One of the most important variables in ensuring a safe oncologic outcome is patient selection and how it relates to margin status. Positive margins on final pathology are potentially complicated by altered architecture. The options for managing positive margins include re-excision or completion mastectomy and reconstruction. The extent of the disease in these situations, especially given the previous generous oncoplastic resection, will often dictate that completion mastectomy is a more appropriate treatment plan. If re-excision is performed, this needs to be done with the reconstructive surgeon. Fortunately, the incidence of positive margins using this approach is felt to be less given the more generous resections. We have demonstrated an average specimen weight over 200 g in oncoplastic resections, compared to about 50 g for non-oncoplastic procedures (**Fig. 6.3**).[8,11] The incidence of positive margins is lower in oncoplastic resections.[12] When completion mastectomy and reconstruction are required, the disadvantages of the reduction procedure are minimal. The benefits of this approach are that (1) no reconstruction options (i.e., flaps) have been used, (2) the contralateral symmetry procedure has already been performed, (3) skin envelope has been reduced, and (4) it is now easier to reconstruct a smaller reduced breast than a large ptotic one (**Fig. 6.4**).

One way to avoid positive margins is to delay reconstruction a few weeks until confirmation of margin status has been obtained (delayed–immediate reconstruction). Most series report a positive margin rate of about 5–10% and, rather than perform an unnecessary second procedure 90–95% of the time, we need to minimize the incidence of positive margins. *Preoperative breast imaging* (i.e., magnetic resonance imaging (MRI), ultrasound or mammography) is helpful in determining the extent of the disease, guiding the necessary resection, and should be employed judiciously when indicated. An imaging study showed that tumor size was underestimated 14% by mammography and 18% by ultrasound, whereas MRI showed no difference when compared to the pathological specimen.[13] *Separate cavity margins* sent at the time of lumpectomy significantly reduces the need for re-excision. Cao demonstrated that final margin status was negative in 60% of patients with positive margins on

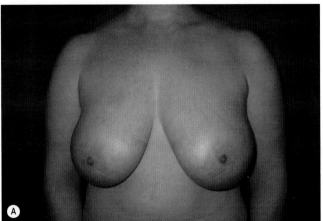

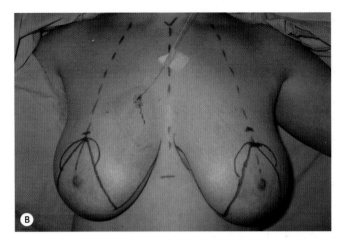

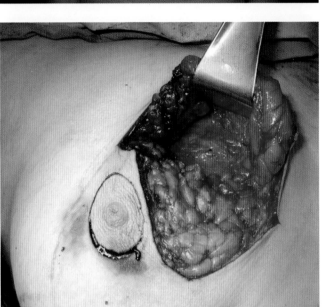

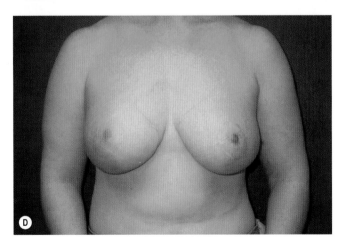

Figure 6.1 This is a 33-year-old woman with stage III breast cancer, who had an excellent response to preoperative chemotherapy and desired breast conservation. In order to minimize the potential for a poor cosmetic result with a defect in the upper pole, she underwent a right wire-guided lumpectomy (100 g) with simultaneous bilateral breast reduction (total volume 250 g left, and 150 g right). The nipple was moved on an inferiorly based dermatoglandular pedicle with the central attachments intact, and used in part to fill the upper pole volume void. Her result is shown at 1 year following completion of right breast radiation therapy.

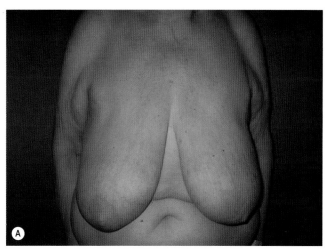
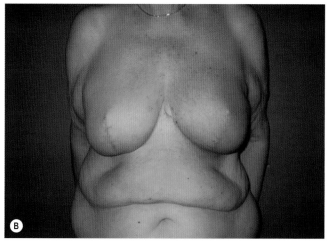

Figure 6.2 This is a 65-year-old woman with subareolar invasive ductal carcinoma. She is not an ideal candidate for skin-sparing mastectomy and breast reconstruction given her body habitus, yet her wishes were for breast reconstruction and symmetry. An alternative option was for her to undergo partial mastectomy and bilateral breast reduction. She had a 150 g lumpectomy including resection of the nipple–areolar complex, followed by bilateral breast reduction. She is shown 1 year following left breast irradiation and deferred nipple reconstruction. Her breasts are soft, sentate and symmetric, which would have been more difficult to obtain following total mastectomy. (Losken A et al. Partial breast reconstruction. *Plast Reconstr Surg* 2008.)

initial resection.[14] Additional intraoperative confirmatory procedures include radiography of the specimen, and intraoperative frozen sections for invasive cancer. *Patient selection* is another important consideration. A recent series has demonstrated a higher rate of positive margins in women under the age of 40 years with extensive ductal carcinoma in situ (DCIS), suggesting delayed immediate reconstruction in those situations.[8] Other patients with potentially difficult margin issues include prior chemotherapy, infiltrating lobular carcinoma, and multicentric disease. In these patients and in any other patient where there is intraoperative concern regarding margin status, the reconstruction should be delayed until margin status has been confirmed.

Operative approach

Steps

1. Patient selection.
2. Preoperative planning.
3. Tumor resection.
4. Reconstruction.

There are four steps to the operative approach. The first is *patient selection*, which has been discussed above. Once it has been established that the patient is a candidate for an oncoplastic reduction, the *preoperative planning* phase can begin. If this is being performed by a two-team approach, then it is crucial that communication exists between the teams. They should review the radiographic imaging, and discuss the anticipated defect location and defect size. This will assist with determination of the most appropriate glandular pedicle required to maintain nipple viability and reshape the mound. Always have a back-up

plan, as occasionally the defect is different from that anticipated, and an alternative approach is required. The patient is marked preoperatively on both sides using relatively conservative markings. If a Wise pattern is drawn, vertical limbs are slightly longer than normal, and the angle is smaller (to ensure minimal tension on the incisions and reduce the potential for healing problems). If radiographically placed wires are being used for the lumpectomy, these should be examined and films reviewed. The combined team should discuss possible access incisions on the mound for tumor resection. Poorly placed incisions could interfere with viability of skin flaps and worsen results.

Tumor resection is then performed through or within Wise patterns if possible, with attention to blood supply and nipple viability. The specimen is weighed to assist with determination of resection goals on the contralateral side. Intraoperative margin assessment could include radiographical imaging, macroscopic assessment, frozen section, or touch cytology. Once separate cavity samples are sent to pathology, the cavity is clipped for postoperative surveillance and guidance for radiation boosts to the tumor bed if required.

Partial mastectomy *reconstruction* is initiated by examining the defect in terms of size and location. It is important to examine the remaining breast tissue and to determine where it is in relation to the defect, the nipple, and the breast mound.

Reconstructive goals are as follows:

1. Keep the nipple alive and position it appropriately on the mound.
2. Fill the dead space.
3. Resect excess breast tissue when necessary.
4. Reshape the breast mound using the pedicles and remaining breast tissue.

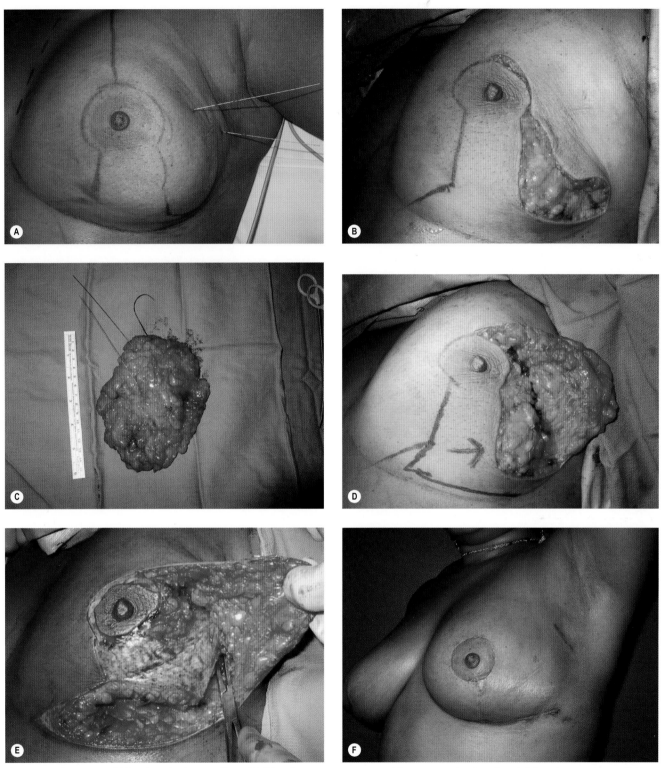

Figure 6.3 This 44-year-old female with a history of lateral DCIS underwent a 110 gram partial mastectomy leaving a lateral defect down to chest wall. Her breast was moderately sized with minimal ptosis. The defect in relation to her breast mound was such that the volume void was lateral. The nipple was in decent position requiring only minimal elevation, and the remaining breast required a lower pole reduction in order to reshape the mound. There was no lateral tissue available to fill the defect. We elected to use a superomedial pedicle and rotate the pedicle as an extended autoaugmentation flap to move the nipple up, fill the lateral defect and reshape the breast mound. This approach was determined after evaluation of the defect, the residual breast tissue and both of these factors in relation to the nipple position and the proposed nipple position. A 118 gram superomedial mastopexy was performed on the contralateral side. (Losken A et al. Partial breast reconstruction. *Plast Reconstr Surg* 2008.)

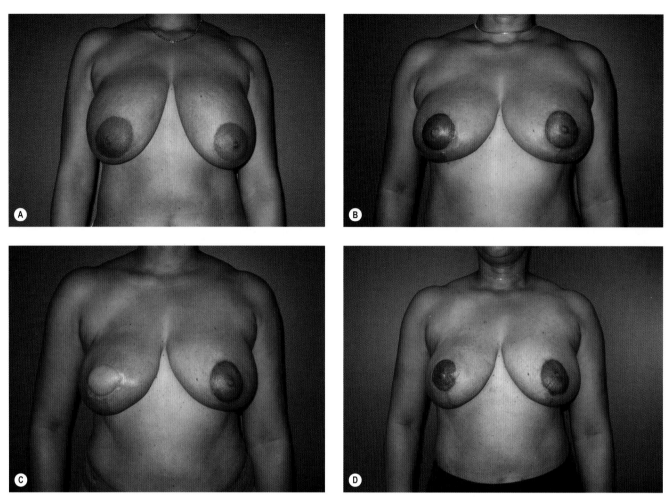

Figure 6.4 This is a 44-year-old woman with macromastia and a history of DCIS who was scheduled to undergo a partial mastectomy. She underwent the partial mastectomy, leaving a defect in the lateral quadrant extending into the subareolar location (**B**). Margin status was confirmed negative, and she was reconstructed a week later using a superomedial pedicle reduction on both sides (**C**). The weight of the partial mastectomy specimen was 80 g, with an additional 218 g resected with the reduction. The contralateral reduction specimen weighed 453 g. Her result is shown following oncoplastic reduction; however, additional DCIS was found within the extra reduction tissue sent. She subsequently had a completion mastectomy and latissimus dorsi flap reconstruction with an implant (**D**).

The first decision is *how to keep the nipple alive*. Typically the shortest pedicle will maximize nipple viability, and allow additional glandular manipulation without worrying about nipple compromise. Many options exist for nipple pedicles, and most surgeons have a favorite. For example, if the superomedial pedicle is your procedure of choice for standard breast reductions, then this technique could be employed for most oncoplastic defects if the patient is a candidate, as long as the defect location is not medial to the nipple. As a general rule, if the pedicle points to or can be rotated into the defect, it can be used. Occasionally it is not possible to preserve the nipple, either because of the size of the breasts, or the location of the tumor. Options include amputation and free nipple graft, or nipple reconstruction at a later date.

Once a decision has been made on nipple preservation, the pedicle is de-epithelialized and dissected with a cautery unit sufficient to allow rotation into the proposed nipple position. *The second decision then is how to fill the dead space*. At this point glandular resection has not yet been performed. If the defect is removed as part of a reduction specimen, and is adequately filled through glandular displacement with the pedicle, and/or remaining glandular tissue, then autoaugmentation is not required. If it is felt that additional glandular flaps are required to fill the dead space, as determined above, then a decision is made based on what tissue is available, and where it is in relation to the nipple pedicle. If the defect can be filled by rotating an extended portion of the original nipple pedicle, this is often the technique of choice. This *single-pedicle autoaugmentation approach* works well for smaller defects in women with smaller or moderate-sized breasts, or when tissue can be taken with the pedicle from a less cosmetically sensitive area and rotated to fill a defect. Another alternative in larger defects in women with large breasts is to fill the dead space with a *secondary pedicle autoaugmentation approach* if the primary pedicle or residual parenchyma is not sufficient. Two pedicles are often safer and will often reduce the length of each respective pedicle, subsequently minimizing the potential for fat necrosis, and maximize the ability to safely manipulate the glandular flaps. The other reason why an additional pedicle is often useful is that the primary nipple pedicle is limited in its range of motion, as the position of the nipple on the breast mound will dictate where that pedicle needs to be. Once it has been determined how to fill the dead space and reshape a breast mound, the *excess dermatoglandular tissue can then be resected*. The weight of the specimen is then added to this additional resection, calculating a total weight for that side. This is useful in trying to keep the ipsilateral breast larger. The *breast mound shaping* is then performed using the glandular pedicles and remaining breast tissue. Glandular shaping is performed using resorbable sutures where necessary, and the skin is then redraped over the mound. Drains are used if the defect is in communication with the axillary dissection.

Skin pattern

The Wise pattern markings are more versatile and allow easy access to tumor location anywhere within the breast mound. They also give more options to reconstruct the defect using glandular flaps. If it is unclear whether glandular flaps will be required to reconstruct the defect, the standard Wise flaps can be elevated about 1 inch thick up to the chest wall without resecting any additional breast tissue or skin. Numerous options will then exist for either primary or secondary pedicles to keep the nipple alive or fill the defect with the skin flaps, then redraped over the mound to complete the reconstruction. The vertical type reduction or mastopexy is useful for smaller breasts, when the defect can be easily accessed through this approach.

Contralateral breast

Management of the contralateral breast is typically performed using a similar technique to that used on the ipsilateral side to maximize symmetry. If an inferior pedicle was used on the involved breasts, an inferior pedicle is often chosen on the contralateral side. Since the ipsilateral side involves a volume loss procedure (partial mastectomy), glandular resection is always required on the opposite breast, even if a mastopexy technique was used for partial breast reconstruction. The contralateral side is purposely kept about 10% smaller than the ipsilateral breast to allow for anticipated radiation fibrosis (**Fig. 6.5**). My preference is to perform the contralateral procedure at the time of resection. If minor changes in shape and size of the contralateral side are required years after radiation therapy these 'fine-tuning' procedures are easier and more predictable than doing the full reduction at that time, which might then require additional revisions to maximize symmetry (**Fig. 6.6**). Other options include doing the opposite breast following breast irradiation, which then would commit everyone to a second procedure, and is often unnecessary since the contralateral revision rate when done simultaneously is only about 5–10%. It is important that the contralateral breast tissue be sent to pathology given the 2–5% incidence of synchronous breast cancer being diagnosed on that side in women with breast cancer.

Reconstruction by defect location

Defect location and size are important determinants in choosing the type of reconstruction to be performed. For simplicity, the defect location will be divided into central, medial, lateral, inner, and outer. The various principles adopted using these techniques are essentially the same for every case. What is different are the nuances in pedicle design and technique, which other than breast and tumor size are determined mainly by tumor location. Lumpectomy type defects in any location can usually be reconstructed using this technique, as long as sufficient breast parenchyma remains. When skin resection is required, then this must be within the Wise pattern reduction specimen, otherwise a local flap reconstruction would be a more appropriate choice.

Lower quadrant tumors in women with larger breasts are ideally suited for the oncoplastic approach. Quadrantectomy type resections are possible, removing skin and parenchyma from this location, reshaping the breast using a superior or superomedial pedicle. Lower pole tumors in moderate-sized breasts can be excised along with skin as needed in the usual vertical pattern, utilizing a superior pedicle followed by plication of the vertical pillars, and vertical reduction on the contralateral side. *Upper quadrant tumors* can be filled as long as the defect is under the skin. Autoaugmentation techniques have become popular to fill the dead space and maintain shape. Inferior, medial, or central pedicles allow for safe excisions in the upper half of the breast without impairing nipple viability. When skin is resected in the upper half of the breast, such remodeling techniques are not possible.

Lateral or upper outer quadrant defects allow parenchymal remodeling using the superomedial pedicle or inferior pedicle. Upper outer quadrant defects can be more difficult to reconstruct when insufficient residual breast tissue is present in that location to fill the defect. In women with medium-sized ptotic breasts and moderate volume void in the upper outer quadrant, the superomedial pedicle can be extended down to the inframammary fold as an autoaugmented pedicle. This can then be rotated to fill a lateral volume void. The vertical pillars are then plicated in the usual fashion to maintain shape.

Medial defects are often reconstructed using inferior lateral or central type pedicles. When the defect is above the proposed Wise pattern markings, the remaining breast parenchyma below the markings is preserved and used to fill the defect. Any contour irregularities in the medial quadrant significantly affect shape and need to be avoided.

Central tumors have in the past been considered a relative contraindication to BCT; however, with the oncoplas-

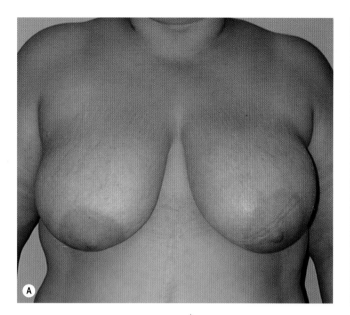

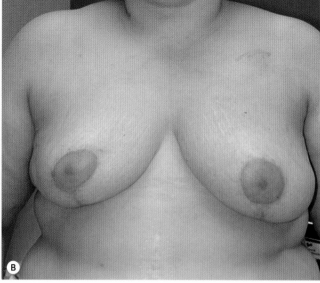

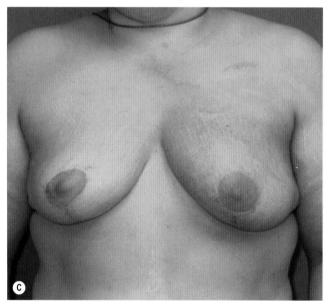

Figure 6.5 This is a 49-year-old woman with a left stage I ductal carcinoma in the inner quadrant (**A**) who underwent a 195 g resection with immediate reduction reconstruction removing 502 g (including lumpectomy) from the left and 536 g from the right. The left breast is larger immediately postoperatively (**B**), with improvement at 2 years following radiation therapy (**C**). (Losken et al. *Ann Plast Surg* 59(3), 2007.)

tic approach in women with macromastia the tumor and nipple–areolar complex can be widely excised and reconstructed using a variety of techniques (**Fig. 6.7**).[15,16] The mound can be remodeled in the inverted T-closure pattern, similar to breast amputation reduction techniques (Fig 6.2). The nipple is then reconstructed later using the reconstruction technique of choice. When the nipple is spared, it can be replaced as a free nipple graft following reconstruction of the mound. Another option if the tumor is located more superiorly or laterally is to perform a central elliptical excision of skin, nipple and parenchyma, and mirror image contralateral reduction for symmetry. A third option includes creation of a skin island on a dermatoglandular pedicle to rotate into the central defect to allow for shape preservation and nipple reconstruction. The breast is marked preoperatively for an inverted T or a vertical approach depending on breast

size, and the skin island is brought in from inferior or medial.

Outcome

Local recurrence is an important outcome measure; however, longer-term studies are required before any definitive conclusions can be made regarding tumor recurrence and survival. It has been proposed that local recurrence would be less given the ability to widely excise the tumor. Studies on partial breast reconstruction are typically small, often lack oncologic outcomes, and long-term results are not available.[17] This review of the literature found that on intermediate follow-up (up to 4.5 years) local recurrence rates varied from 0 to 1.8% per year, and cosmetic failure rates varied from 0 to 18%.

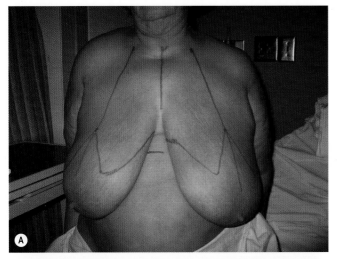

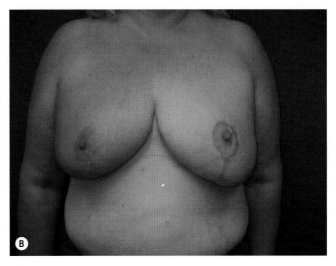

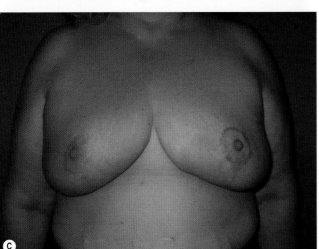

Figure 6.6 This 49-year-old female with right-sided invasive ductal carcinoma in the upper outer quadrant underwent partial mastectomy (biopsy weight 244 g) followed by a bilateral central mound breast reduction (total weight 523 g on the right and 596 g on the left). She is shown 2 years following right-sided breast irradiation with some breast asymmetry. Since the right breast had preservation of shape, a small lower pole reduction was performed on the left side to improve her shape and symmetry.

Clough demonstrated an actuarial 5-year local recurrence rate using this technique of 9.4 %.[18] Another series of 70 patients who underwent oncoplastic surgery for breast cancer demonstrated an actuarial 5-year local recurrence rate of 8.5%.[19]

Postoperative *surveillance* is also important in this patient population and in order for this approach to be deemed safe we need to demonstrate that it does not interfere with our ability to detect recurrence. One concern has been that the additional surgery and tissue rearrangement of breast tissue could potentially alter the architecture and influence the pattern of recurrence or ability to screen accurately. Surgical clips at the tumor margin will identify the tumor bed to assist with radiation boosts, postoperative surveillance and re-exploration, if necessary. We have recently compared mammographic changes and surveillance in women with BCT alone versus those with oncoplastic reductions, and found no interference in the accuracy of post-surveillance.[20] The other question we had was whether the combined procedure delayed the concept of mammographic stabilization or reduced the sensitivity of this screening tool. There was a slight trend toward longer times to mammographic stabilization in the study group (21.2 months for BCT vs 25.6 months for oncoplastic, $p = 0.23$), which is expected given the additional scarring, inflammation, and parenchymal alteration associated with the reconstruction. This time to mammographic stability in the oncoplastic group demonstrated a 95% confidence interval between 20 and 30 months. Parenchymal density was similar in both groups, suggesting that the sensitivity of mammography was not affected. This suggests longer than 6 months' screening is necessary in these patients, possibly until about 2.5–3 years. Additional tissue sampling (fine-needle aspiration, core biopsy, etc.) is often required given the nature of these combined procedures, and the importance of ruling out tumor recurrence. These issues all need to be discussed with the patient preoperatively, as well as with the multi-disciplinary team.

Local *wound healing complications* include delayed healing, skin necrosis, infection, and wound dehiscence; however, these are usually minimal and do not delay the initiation of neoadjuvant therapy. Most series have demonstrated excellent patient and surgeon satisfaction with the cosmetic results using these techniques; however,

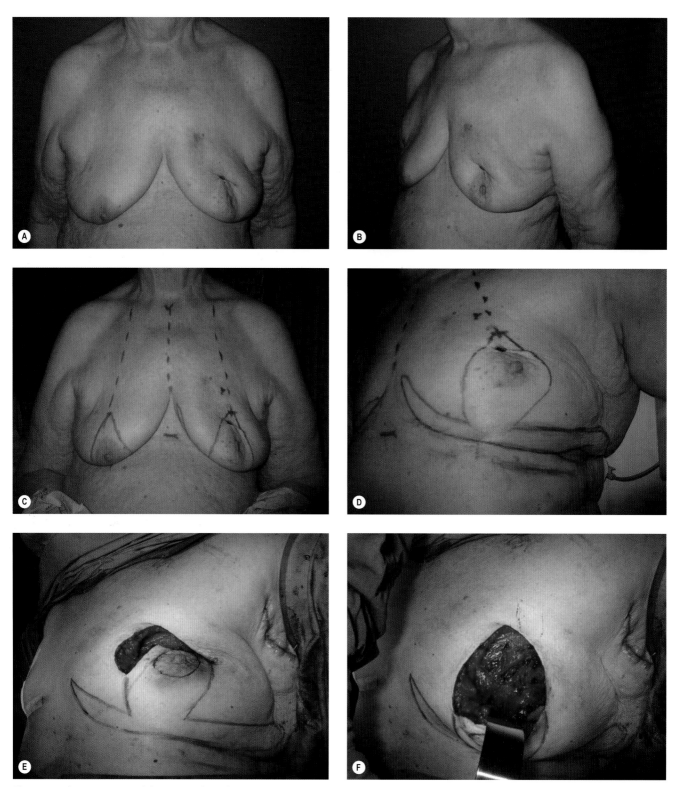

Figure 6.7 This is an 80-year-old woman with small ptotic breasts who had a left-sided carcinoma arising in an adenomyoepithelioma. She already had a lumpectomy with positive margins, and a deformity above the nipple. Mastectomy and reconstruction would have been difficult given her age and breast shape. She had a 60 g re-excision, leaving a defect above and beneath the nipple. The nipple was essentially flat on the chest wall following resection, without any tissue above to fill the void. We used the medial and lateral dermatoglandular flaps in a rotation fashion to place beneath and above the nipple, demonstrating decent shape and nipple projection at the completion of the case. A small central mound contralateral reduction was performed. She is shown 6 months following completion of left-sided breast irradiation. (Losken A. *Oncoplastic Breast Surgery*. Quality Medical Publishing, St Louis, MO.)

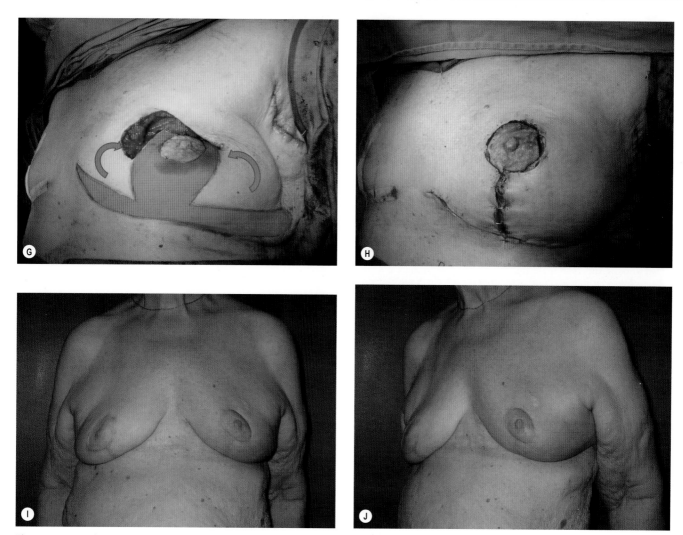

Figure 6.7, cont'd

Table 6.2 Partial mastectomy reconstruction using reduction techniques

Author	No. cases	Complications (%)	Cosmetic result/ patient satisfaction (good–excellent)	Local recurrence (%)	Follow-up (months)
Losken 2007	63	22	95	2	40
Clough 2003	101	20	88	7	46
Munhoz 2006	74	17	93	0	22
Goffman 2005	55	NR	72	13[a]	18
Chang 2004	37	19	70	0	
Kronowitz 2008	33	24	NR	7	36

[a]High percentage of T3, T4 tumors.
NR, not reported.

longer-term outcomes will be interesting, especially given the persistent effects of radiation with time. Breast shape is typically preserved with time, although some radiation fibrosis can be encountered. In these situations it is relatively easy to reduce the contralateral breast further than to reconstruct a radiated deformity.

Another important outcome measure is *patient satisfaction*. A limited group of women in our series report an acceptable aesthetic result in 95% of cases at 6 months' follow-up (**Table 6.2**). Although this is relatively short follow-up, patients are generally pleased with their results. Longer-term follow-up is crucial, especially given the effects of radiation therapy on breast shape with time. Other series have reported favorable aesthetic results and patient satisfaction with this approach.[21–23]

Conclusions

The immediate reconstruction of partial mastectomy defects using mammaplasty reduction or mastopexy techniques is both safe and effective in appropriately selected patients. Its popularity will likely continue to increase given the increased demand for breast conservation and the decreased tolerance for poor cosmetic results. This technique is often the preferred approach given its relative simplicity and predictability, especially in women with macromastia, where mastectomy and reconstruction are often more difficult, with higher morbidity and worse cosmetic results. More stringent patient selection and attention to tumor resection will minimize the incidence of positive margins and improve outcome. This approach broadens the indications for BCT, preserves symmetry and shape, and maintains patients' satisfaction while maintaining successful oncologic outcome and cancer surveillance.

References

1. Fisher B, Anderson S, Bryant J, et al. Twenty-year follow up of a randomized trial comparing total mastectomy, lumpectomy, and lumpectomy plus irradiation of the treatment of invasive breast cancer. N Eng J Med 2002; 347:1233–1241.
2. Veronesi U, Casinelly N, Mariani L, et al. Twenty-year follow-up of a randomized study comparing breast conserving surgery with radical mastectomy for early breast cancer. N Eng J Med 2002; 347:1227–1232.
3. Gray JR, McCormick B, Cox L, et al. Primary breast irradiation in large-breasted or heavy women: analysis of cosmetic outcome. Int J Radiat Oncol Biol Phys 1991; 21:347–354.
4. Zierhut D, Flentje M, Frank C, et al. Conservative treatment of breast cancer: modified irradiation technique for women with large breasts. Radiother Oncol 1994; 31:256–261.
5. Brierly JD, Paterson ICM, Lallemand RC, et al. The influence of breast size on late radiation reaction following excision and radiotherapy for early breast cancer. Clin Oncol 1991; 3:6–9.
6. Clark K, Le MG, Sarrazin D, et al. Analysis of locoregional relapse in patients with early breast cancer treated by excision and radiotherapy: experience of the Institute Gustave-Roussy. Int J Radiat Oncol Biol Phys 1985; 11:137–145.
7. Clough KB, Nos C, Salmon RJ, et al. Conservative treatment of breast cancer by mammaplasty and irradiation: a new approach to lower quadrant tumors. Plast Reconstr Surg 1995; 96(2):363–370.
8. Losken A, Styblo TM, Carlson GW, et al. Management algorithm and outcome evaluation of partial mastectomy defects treated using reduction or mastopexy techniques. Ann Plast Surg 2007; 59(3):235.
9. Munhoz AM, Montag E, Arruda EG, et al. Critical analysis of reduction mammaplasty techniques in combination with conservative breast surgery for early breast cancer treatment. Plast Reconstr Surg 2006; 117(4):1091–1103.
10. Spear SL, Burke JB, Forman D, et al. Experience with reduction mammaplasty following breast conservation surgery and radiation therapy. Plast Reconstr Surg 1998; 102(6):1913–1916.
11. Clough KB, Lewis JS, Couturaud B, et al. Oncoplastic techniques allow extensive resections for breast-conserving therapy of breast cancer. Ann Surg 2003; 237(1):26–34.
12. Kaur N, Petit JY, Rietjens M, et al. Comparative study of surgical margins in oncoplastic surgery and quadrantectomy in breast cancer. Ann Surg Oncol 2005; 12(7):539–545.
13. Boetes C, Mus RD, Holland R, et al. Breast tumors: comparative accuracy of MR imaging relative to mammography and US for demonstrating extent, Radiology 1995; 197:743–747.
14. Cao D, Lin C, Woo SH, et al. Separate cavity margin sampling at the time of initial breast lumpectomy significantly reduces the need for re-excision. Am J Surg Pathol 2005; 29(12):1625–1632.
15. Chung TL, Schnaper L, Silverman R, et al. A novel reconstructive technique following central lumpectomy. Plast Reconstr Surg 2006; 118(1):23–27.
16. McCulley SJ, Dourani P, Macmillan RD. Therapeutic mammaplasty for centrally located breast tumors. Plast Reconstr Surg 2006; 117(2):366–373.
17. Asgeursson KS, Rasheed T, McCulley SJ, et al. Oncological and cosmetic outcomes of oncoplastic breast conserving surgery. Eur J Surg Oncol 2005; 31(8):817–823.
18. Clough KB, Lewis JS, Couturaud B, et al. Oncoplastic techniques allow extensive resections for breast-conserving therapy of breast cancer. Ann Surg 2003; 237(1):26–34.
19. Cothier-Savey I, Otmezguine Y, Calitchi E, et al. [Value of reduction mammoplasty in the conservative treatment of breast neoplasm. Apropos of 70 cases]. Ann Chir Plast Esthet 1996; 41:346–353.
20. Schaefer TG, Losken A, Newell MS, et al. The impact of oncoplastic breast reduction on postoperative cancer surveillance (in press).
21. Goffman TE, Schneider H, Hay K, Cosmesis with bilateral mammoreduction for conservative breast cancer treatment. Breast J 2005; 11(3):195–198.
22. Chang E, Johnson N, Webber B. Bilateral reduction mammoplasty in combination with lumpectomy for treatment of breast cancer in patients with macromastia Am J Surg 2004; 187(5):647–650; discussion 650–651.
23. Kronowitz SJ, Hunt KK, Kuerer HM, et al. Practical guidelines for repair of partial mastectomy defects using the breast reduction technique in patients undergoing breast conservation therapy. Plast Reconstr Surg 2007; 120(7):1755–1768.

Lateral Thoracic Flaps in Breast Reconstruction

Joshua L Levine • P Pravin Reddy • Robert J Allen

Introduction

In this chapter, we present the use of lateral thoracic skin and subcutaneous tissues as an option for partial breast reconstruction. Lateral thoracic skin and fat are an excellent source of tissue for reconstruction of partial mastectomy defects (after lumpectomy), as well as for augmenting both reconstructed and normal breasts for the purpose of achieving symmetry. The donor site is well concealed and may even serve to improve the lateral chest wall contour. Tissue is harvested on one of three different pedicles, leaving the latissimus dorsi (LD) muscle intact. We find the flaps to be reliable and the technique reproducible, offering an excellent alternative to fat grafting, prostheses, and the LD flap.

Secondary defects in breast reconstruction

The post-mastectomy defect is frequently treated with autologous breast reconstruction. Despite being unrivaled in restoring symmetry, ptosis, and texture to the reconstructed breast, many patients undergoing reconstruction require secondary or revision procedures in order to achieve symmetry, an acceptable final volume, or to simply correct contour irregularities.[1]

Patients with early-stage breast cancer are increasingly treated with breast conservation therapy. Treatment may comprise lumpectomy and sentinel lymph node dissection with or without axillary node clearance and radiation therapy.[2] However, breast conservation therapy is known to result in a variety of contour irregularities which pose difficult reconstructive challenges. It is widely accepted that between 20% and 30% of patients undergoing breast conservation therapy experience poor or mediocre cosmetic outcomes as a direct result of lumpectomy and radiation fibrosis.[3] An estimated 71% of patients seek treatment for correction of partial mastectomy defects and contour deformities.[4] Often, these defects present the surgeon with a greater reconstructive challenge when compared with reconstruction of a defect resulting from a total mastectomy.

The need for more volume in a reconstructed breast also arises when a reconstructed breast needs to be revised, for example by removal of fat necrosis. This can result in a reconstruction that is smaller than the contralateral breast. Another situation requiring augmentation of volume is when a reconstructed breast is larger than the contralateral normal breast. Lateral thoracic flaps can be used to correct all the aforementioned problems.

Many partial mastectomy defects require only moderate amounts of volume in order to achieve satisfactory correction. While the LD flap has long been the workhorse in transferring autologous tissue to the breast mound in order to reconstruct partial defects, it exacts a high price on the patient. Sacrifice of the LD muscle results in early fatigue with repetitive arm extension as well as weak internal/external rotation of the upper extremity.[5] Since the advent of perforator flaps, it is possible to create muscle-sparing flaps utilizing the lateral thoracic and axillary tissue. Furthermore, the LD flap harvest site is prone to the complication of seroma formation.

An alternative to the myocutaneous LD flap is to simply utilize the lateral thoracic and axillary skin and subcutaneous tissues, based on the perforating blood vessels that supply them. The thoracic skin and fat immediately lateral to the breast provides a logical source for tissue with which to reconstruct the adjacent breast (**Table 7.1**). Lateral thoracic skin is similar in color and texture to native breast and offers an excellent match. Furthermore, it is possible to harvest large amounts of skin and subcutaneous tissue without violating muscle. Lateral thoracic skin may be applied to breast reconstruction in conjunction with an implant when necessary. The indications and contraindications for use of lateral thoracic flaps are listed in **Tables 7.2** and **7.3**.

In many patients the lateral thoracic and axillary skin are present as an unsightly bulge or roll. Harvest of skin from this area provides the additional potential advantage of improving the contour of the lateral chest wall. Harvest of lateral thoracic skin necessarily results in an additional surgical scar; however, the scar is strategically positioned under the arm at the level of the bra line. Thus the donor site is effectively camouflaged in a manner cosmetically acceptable to both the patient and surgeon.

Preoperative history and considerations

The first consideration is the amount of volume of tissue available. The 'pinch test' will help to determine the amount of tissue available. The surgeon must ascertain that a flap of width 7–9 cm is available for harvest with enough subcutaneous fat to provide the volume required. Extensive axillary surgery may be a contraindication to use of the lateral thoracic tissue. If the patient has had an axillary node dissection, it is necessary to review the operative report so that the surgeon knows that the thoracodorsal artery and vein are intact for use as a thoracodorsal artery perforator (TDAP) (Angrigiani) flap.[6] If this cannot be ascertained, a Doppler signal in the appropriate position at the anterior axillary line may represent either an intercostal perforator or a direct cutaneous branch from the axillary artery. Any of these may be pedicle options, and the choice may influence the degree of flap mobility and rotation. Previous implant reconstruction can also sometimes disrupt normal anatomy in the anterior axillary line, rendering intercostal perforators unavailable for use. Liposuction to the lateral thorax is a contraindication to the use of this tissue, and radiation therapy often causes skin changes that limit the skin's availability.

Flap design

The flap is designed with the patient in the upright position. It is important to mark the patient prior to positioning on the operating table as this provides the surgeon with the opportunity to assess lateral thoracic bulge. Immediately posterior to the lateral breast at the anterior axillary line a handheld 8 MHz Doppler is used to locate signals at the anterior edge of the LD. Signals in this area can be either perforators off of the thoracodorsal, a direct cutaneous branch from the axillary artery, or an intercostal perforator. One, two or three appropriately placed signals are selected and the flap is designed around them. The anterior apex of the flap is adjacent to the lateral breast or breast flap. The flap is oriented horizontally within the bra line as an ellipse with a width of 7–10 cm and length of 15–20 cm (**Fig. 7.1**).

Relevant anatomy and operative approach

The thoracodorsal artery flap (TDAP)

The TDAP flap represents an adipocutaneous flap supplied by perforating vessels of the thoracodorsal artery. Originally described in 1994, the TDAP was initially applied to forearm and chest reconstruction.[6] The TDAP accomplishes the same reconstructive goals as the LD flap, with the notable advantage that the important LD muscle is completely preserved.[7]

Table 7.1 Advantages of lateral thoracic flaps in breast reconstruction

Excellent skin and tissue match with native breast
Convenient source of volume
Scar easily concealed under the arm within the bra line
Minimal donor site morbidity
No sacrifice of muscle
Reduced incidence of seroma when compared with LD flaps
Improved thoracic wall contour as a result of elimination of lateral roll/bulge

---

Table 7.2 Indications for lateral thoracic and axillary flap breast reconstruction

Correction of partial mastectomy defects
Correction of contour irregularities
Augmenting volume of reconstructed breast mound
Augmenting volume of normal contralateral breast for symmetry

---

Table 7.3 Contraindications to lateral thoracic and axillary flap breast reconstruction

Previous surgery to lateral chest wall
Posterolateral thoracotomy
Patient preference

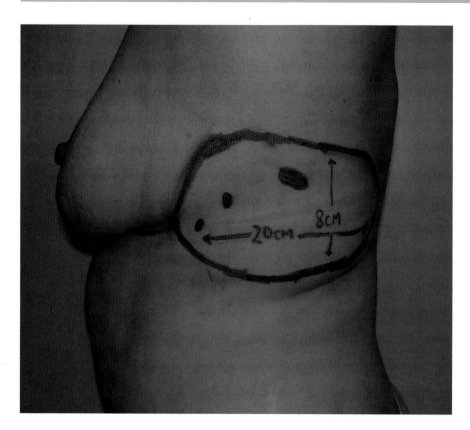

Figure 7.1 Marking of the lateral thoracic flap is demonstrated with the patient in the upright position. This is of importance as the lateral bulge can be best evaluated with the patient standing. Candidate perforators are identified with the hand-held Doppler and marked. We recommend that flap width not exceed 8 cm in width as illustrated.

An algorithm for the selection of a pedicle for the transfer of lateral thoracic tissue has previously been detailed by Levine.[8] The thoracodorsal artery takes origin from the subscapular artery, descending along the lateral and deep surface of the LD muscle. Along its course the thoracodorsal artery gives off the serratus branch before terminating in anterior and posterior branches. The anterior and posterior branches yield equal numbers of perforators to supply the overlying skin of the lateral chest wall. A large skin paddle may be designed over any one of the perforators of adequate caliber.

The patient is placed on the operating room table in the supine position, with a bolster under the ipsilateral chest. The ipsilateral arm is prepped into the field with the use of a stockinet cover (**Fig. 7.2**). Beveling is used to maximize the amount of subcutaneous fat harvested. The flap is elevated from posterior to anterior at the level of the latissimus fascia. When a vessel is encountered it is evaluated for suitability in terms of its size. When an appropriate vessel is selected, the dissection is continued down through the LD. The muscle fibers are gently separated, while preserving the anterior edge of the muscle. When the dissection reaches the thoracodorsal artery and vein, great care must be taken to preserve the thoracodorsal nerve. The dissection continues superiorly toward the axillary vessels; the longer the pedicle dissection, the greater the arc of rotation. The anterior edge of LD must be separated for a sufficient length to enable the flap to be passed through (**Figs 7.3** and **7.4**). The flap is then placed either behind the breast or reconstructed breast, or used to fill in a contour defect.

Case example

A 45-year-old woman with ductal carcinoma in situ (DCIS) of the right breast presented for mastectomy and deep inferior epigastric artery perforator (DIEP) breast reconstruction. The mastectomy weight of 410 g was replaced with a DIEP flap that weighed 740 g. The resulting reconstructed breast was made larger than the normal contralateral breast with the plan of reducing it at a second-stage nipple procedure. However, when the patient came back for her second stage, she decided that the larger volume was more appropriate for her, and that she would prefer augmentation of the normal breast, rather than reduction of the reconstructed breast. She was an excellent candidate for the use of her lateral thoracic tissue for autologous augmentations (**Figs 7.1–7.4** and **Figs 7.5** and **7.6**).

The lateral thoracic flap

The lateral thoracic flap or axillary flap derives axial blood supply in part from one or more direct cutaneous branches from one of three potential source vessels: the lateral thoracic artery; the axillary artery, also known as the accessory lateral thoracic artery; or the thoracodorsal artery. Any of these vessels provides an excellent source on which the axillary flap may be based either as a pedicled or free flap.[9] Reports in the literature as to the consistency of these vessels vary. A single series of 100

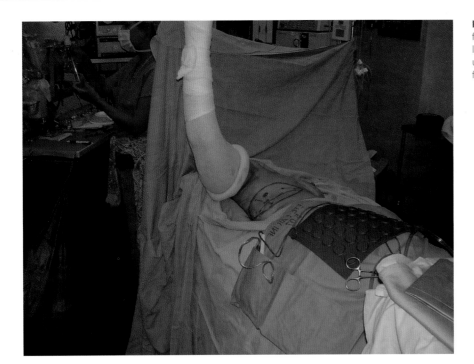

Figure 7.2 Patient positioning in preparation for flap harvest. Note that the patient is in the lateral decubitus position with the ipsilateral upper extremity free-draped into the operative field.

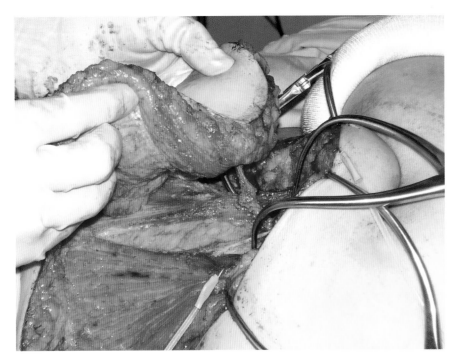

Figure 7.3 The lateral thoracic flap is elevated based on the thoracodorsal artery perforator. Note the muscle fibers of the anterior edge of the latissimus dorsi are separated in order to expose the perforator to its source vessel, as well as to create a portal through which the flap may be delivered to its recipient site under the breast.

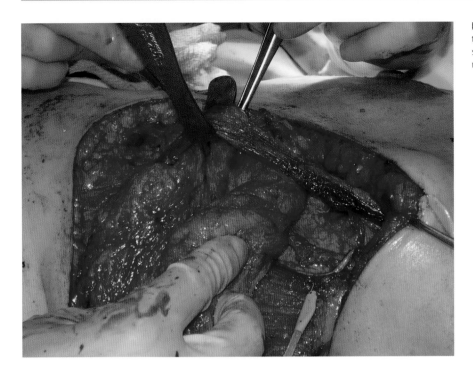

Figure 7.4 The mobilized flap is delivered to the recipient site by passing it through the separated anterior border of the latissimus dorsi muscle.

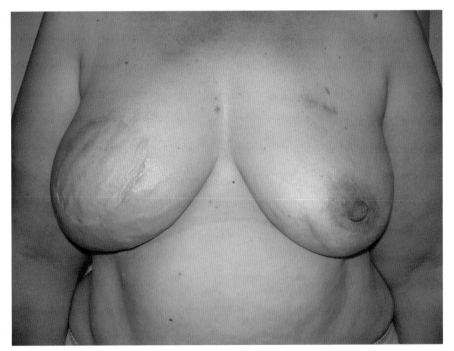

Figure 7.5 Preoperative photograph of a patient demonstrating volume deficiency of the left breast compared with the DIEP reconstructed right breast.

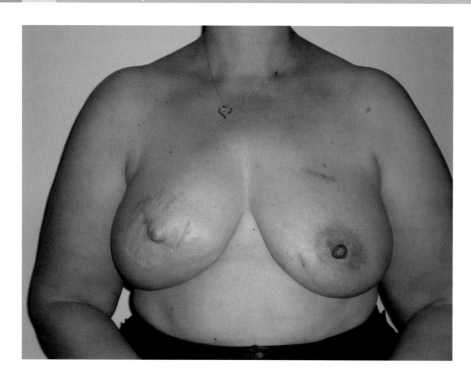

Figure 7.6 Demonstration of the degree of volume correction of the normal breast achieved with the lateral thoracic flap. Note the camouflage of all surgical incisions.

cadaver dissections of the subscapular–thoracodorsal system demonstrated a direct cutaneous branch from the thoracodorsal artery in 47% of specimens, whereas a direct cutaneous branch from the subscapular artery was noted in 7%.[10] A subsequent study by a separate author in 2003 on 20 cadavers concluded a direct cutaneous branch from the thoracodorsal artery in 55% of specimens.[11] Skin and subcutaneous tissue can reliably be transferred to the breast based on one of three direct cutaneous vessels. The source artery may be further mobilized to facilitate transfer of tissue to the defect.

Case example

A 48-year-old woman who had previously undergone lumpectomy, axillary dissection, radiation, and chemotherapy of the right breast for cancer presented with a deformity of the inferior pole of the right breast. A skin paddle extending over the LD muscle was designed as originally described by Holmstrom and Lossing.[12] The base of the flap measured 7 cm and the length 16 cm. Dissection proceeded from lateral to anterior to the level of the anterior axillary line. During the course of the dissection in this case, no thoracodorsal perforators were identified; however, immediately anterior to the edge of the LD muscle, a direct cutaneous branch of the thoracodorsal artery was identified and preserved. This single pedicle adequately perfused the entire flap and was selected as the basis for the flap. The flap was then completely elevated off the underlying muscle. An island flap was created by dividing the medial skin bridge, thus further mobilizing the tissue. Subglandular dissection and scar contracture release led to formation of a pocket to accommodate the flap. The flap was

then de-epithelialized and turned over, following which it was inserted into the submammary pocket in order to reconstruct the inferior pole of the breast mound. A mastopexy was performed on the contralateral breast to achieve symmetry. The patient's postoperative course was unremarkable and no complications were observed.

The intercostal perforator flap

The intercostal perforator flap bases the lateral thoracic skin and subcutaneous tissue on intercostal artery perforators entering the flap base in the anterior axillary line.[13] A large and reliable flap may be created for use as a rotation flap with or without an implant. It may also be applied as a turnover flap to augment deficiencies of the lower pole of the breast.

Case example

A 51-year-old female with a history of left breast DCIS, bilateral mastectomy and pedicled transverse rectus abdominis myocutaneous (TRAM) reconstruction, radiation and subsequent failure of the left TRAM presented for left breast reconstruction (**Fig. 7.7**). She underwent a left inferior gluteal artery perforator (IGAP) reconstruction which lacked projection compared to the right TRAM (**Fig. 7.8**). She was taken back for left reconstruction augmentation with an ICAP flap. The flap was designed and dissected as described. When no thoracodorsal perforators or direct cutaneous branches were encountered, an intercostal perforator was selected and dissected down through the intercostal muscle as far as possible (**Fig. 7.9**). The flap was de-epithelialized and advanced into position

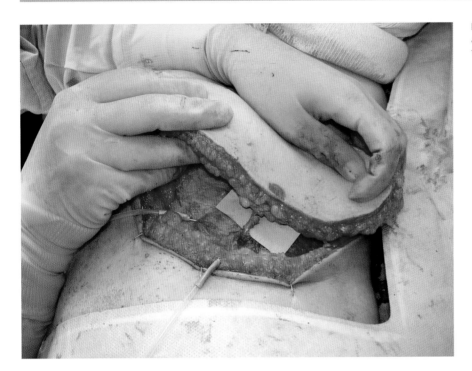

Figure 7.7 Demonstration of the intercostal artery perforator (ICAP) vessel as it emerges from the intercostal muscle.

under the left IGAP, and provided more volume and projection (**Fig. 7.10**).

Systematic approach to application of lateral thoracic and axillary tissue in breast reconstruction

The case examples presented illustrate the variety of options available when using lateral thoracic or axillary skin in breast reconstruction. The vascular anatomy has been well described and forms the basis for selection of an appropriate pedicle and preoperative Doppler planning. **Tables 7.4** and **7.5** list the pearls and pitfalls in the planning of lateral thoracic flaps.

The elliptical flap is designed horizontally with the anterior apex positioned at the anterior axillary line adjacent to the lateral breast flap. The flap measures 6–10 cm in width and 15–20 cm in length. The flap is strategically positioned over Doppler signals obtained prior to marking. The flap curves slightly upward following the contour of the ribs, with the anterior apex extending slightly beyond the LD muscle.

Pedicle option I

The dissection is started posteriorly. Skin and subcutaneous tissues are incised to the level of the LD muscle. Beveling is used to maximize the volume of harvested tissue. The dissection then continues medially in a plane between the LD muscle and overlying fat. With the aid of loupe magnification, the thoracodorsal perforators are identified near the lateral edge of the latissimus dorsi. If the perforators are adequate, they are preserved and dissected through the muscle fibers until the thoracodorsal artery is identified. The thoracodorsal nerve is preserved and separated from the accompanying blood vessel. The flap is then delivered through the opening created in the LD muscle and the thoracodorsal artery dissected until adequate pedicle length is achieved.

Pedicle option II

In cases where the thoracodorsal perforator is deemed inadequate for flap perfusion, the dissection is continued anteriorly. The next logical source of flap perfusion includes the direct cutaneous branches of the axillary, thoracodorsal, or lateral thoracic vessels. When present, direct cutaneous branches confer the added advantage of obviating dissection of the LD muscle. As in the previously described pedicle option I, the cutaneous branch is dissected to its source artery in order to obtain adequate pedicle length.

Pedicle option III

In cases where neither of the first two options is available, then the flap may be based on the intercostal perforator vessels. Intercostal perforators are proven to be consistent and reliable. In patients who have undergone extensive surgery in the lateral thoracic area, the intercostal perforators may not be available. Based on the intercostal perforators, the flap can either be rotated 90 degrees, advanced into position or applied as a turnover flap.

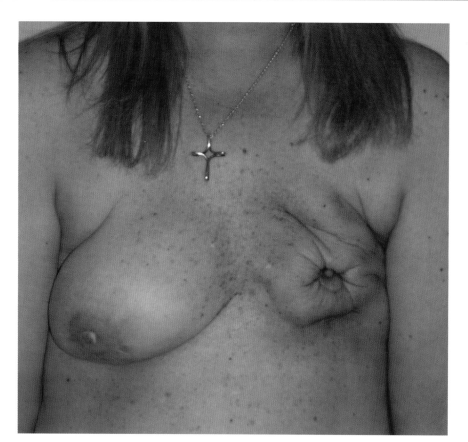

Figure 7.8 After bilateral TRAM with radiation and failure on the left.

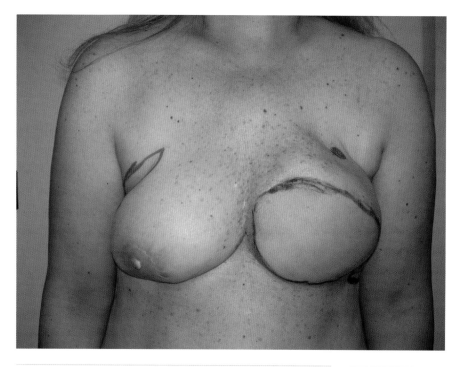

Figure 7.9 IGAP used to replace failed TRAM. Left reconstruction lacks projection and there is a depression superiorly.

Table 7.4 Pearls

Preoperative Doppler identification of candidate vessels
Contingency based on three separate pedicles
Positioning of flap over the appropriate intercostal space
Use of micro-bipolar cautery instrument in perforator dissection
Bevel to obtain more volume

Table 7.5 Pitfalls

History of previous surgery compromising available perforators
Trying to harvest too much skin will make the defect difficult to close
Trying to rotate the flap more than 90 degrees
Not getting enough pedicle length due to timid dissection all the way to
 the axillary vessels

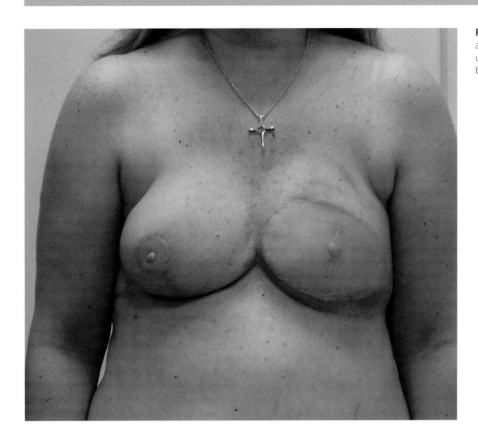

Figure 7.10 Left IGAP reconstruction has been augmented with ICAP to improve volume and upper lateral depression. The right TRAM has been revised.

Optimizing outcomes

Rigorous preoperative planning is essential. This requires thorough knowledge of the vascular anatomy as described and detailed knowledge of the patient's surgical history in the region. Positioning in the operating room is also of vital importance. The patient is bolstered almost to the lateral decubitus position, and the arm is prepped into the field. This way the arm can be moved or hung from an IV pole during the procedure.

Complications

Complications associated with the lateral thoracic flap are related to venous congestion from trying to move the flap too far, or rotating it too much. This can be avoided by continuing the pedicle dissection as far as possible into the axilla. Drains are placed in at the donor site, and seromas have not been an issue.

Post-operative care

Patients undergoing reconstruction of the breast using the lateral thoracic flap are admitted to the hospital overnight. The patient is on restricted activities with limited range of motion of the ipsilateral upper extremity for 24

hours. The flap is usually totally buried, so monitoring is not possible or needed. If a skin island is left temporarily, the flap can be monitored by standard methods. If the flap becomes congested, releasing some sutures or patient repositioning will probably take care of the problem. The patient may resume normal activities by postoperative day two. The patient is discharged home with closed-suction drains which are removed on follow-up, provided the yield is less than 30 cm³ per day.

Conclusions

We present the lateral thoracic skin area as a versatile donor site with a range of possibilities for flap perfusion. The use of lateral thoracic tissue presents the advantage of complete muscle preservation; a cosmetically acceptable donor site scar; and removal of redundant lateral thoracic skin with elimination of a sometimes unsightly roll. The vascular anatomy of the lateral thoracic tissue is well defined and preoperative Doppler interrogation provides the surgeon with several perfusion options. These factors make the lateral thoracic tissue a safe, reliable, and reproducible procedure for reconstruction for a variety of breast reconstruction defects.

References

1. Beahm EK, Walton RL. Revision in autologous breast reconstruction: principles and approach. Clin Plast Surg 2007; 34(1):139–162.
2. Fisher B, Anderson S, Bryant J, et al. Twenty-year follow-up of a randomized trial comparing total mastectomy, lumpectomy, and lumpectomy plus irradiation for the treatment of invasive breast cancer. N Engl J Med. 2002; 347(16):1233–1241.
3. Amichetti M, Busana L, Caffo O. Long-term cosmetic outcome and toxicity in patients treated with quadrantectomy and radiation therapy for early-stage breast cancer. Oncology 1995; 52:177–181.
4. Clough KB, Cuminet J, Fitoussi A, et al. Cosmetic sequelae after conservative treatment for breast cancer: classification and results of surgical correction. Ann Plast Surg 1998; 41:471–481.
5. Spear SL, Hess CL. A review of the biomechanical and functional changes in the shoulder following transfer of the latissimus dorsi muscles. Plast Reconstr Surg 2005; 115(7):2070–2073.
6. Angrigiani C, Grill D, Siebert J. Latissimus dorsi musculocutaneous flap without muscle. Plast Reconstr Surg 1995; 96:1608–1614.
7. Khoobehi K, Allen RJ, Montegut WJ. Thoracodorsal artery perforator flap for reconstruction. 90th Annual Scientific Assembly of the Southern Medical Association, Baltimore, MD, November 20–24. South Med J 1996; 89.
8. Levine JL, Soueid NE, Allen RJ. Algorithm for autologous breast reconstruction for partial mastectomy defects. Plast Reconstr Surg 2005; 116(3):762–767.
9. Harii K, Torii S, Sekiguchi J. The free lateral thoracic flap. Plast Reconstr Surg 1978; 62:212–222.
10. Roswell AR, Davies D, Eisenberg N, et al. The anatomy of the subscapular-thoracodorsal artery arterial system: study of 100 cadaver dissections. Br J Plast Surg 1984; 537:574–576.
11. Guerra AB, Metzinger SE, Lund KM, et al. The thoracodorsal artery perforator flap: clinical experience and anatomic study with emphasis on harvest techniques. Plast Reconstr Surg 2004; 114(1):32–41; discussion 42–43.
12. Holmstrom H, Lossing C. Lateral thoracodorsal flap: an intercostal perforator flap for breast reconstruction. Semin Plast Surg 2002; 16:53–59.
13. Hamdi M, Van Landuyt K, de Frene B, et al. The versatility of the inter-costal artery perforator (ICAP) flaps. J Plast Reconstr Aesthet Surg 2006; 59(6):644–652.

CHAPTER 8

Latissimus Dorsi Flap Repair of the Partial Mastectomy Defect

Neil Fine • Kristina O'Shaughnessy

Introduction

Traditional breast conservation therapy (BCT), consisting of lumpectomy, sentinel lymph node biopsy, possible axillary dissection, and radiation therapy, is medically equivalent to mastectomy with regard to overall long-term survival rates and has been the recommended treatment of choice for women with early-stage breast cancer.[1] BCT has always focused on optimizing cosmetic goals and minimizing the psychological morbidity of a mastectomy, while maintaining low rates of local recurrence. Historically, BCT was only performed when adequate tumor-free margins could be obtained with cosmetically acceptable results. Although large tumor size alone is not considered a contraindication for BCT in terms of local tumor control, it is an important variable in obtaining good cosmetic results.[2] Specifically, the breast volume excised in relation to total breast volume directly correlates with cosmesis and patient satisfaction after BCT. The site of the breast tumor also plays a role in anticipating poor aesthetic outcomes, such that medial tumors lead to more unfavorable cosmesis.[3] Oncoplastic techniques have extended the indications of breast conservation therapy in the modern day management of patients with breast cancer. Combining wide resection of breast parenchyma with simultaneous reconstruction of the defect, oncoplastic breast surgery avoids significant risk of local deformity, thereby preserving aesthetics while increasing the accuracy of local disease control.[4]

The critical factor in achieving an oncologically sound resection is tumor margin clearance.[5] Achieving oncologic clearance with increasing tumor size requires extensive breast volume resection, resulting in large partial mastectomy defects requiring reconstruction using volume displacement or volume replacement techniques. Volume displacement, described in a previous chapter, uses local glandular or dermoglandular rearrangement to fill the resection defect. Depending on the amount of breast volume resected, a simultaneous contralateral reduction may be required to achieve symmetry. Surgical resection ultimately reaches a maximum volume limit when volume displacement techniques will not be adequate to achieve an aesthetically pleasing result, even if the contralateral breast is reduced for symmetry.[6] In these cases, volume replacement techniques are necessary to restore breast shape and contour. These techniques use autologous tissue to replace the volume of excised breast parenchyma. As the volume is restored, contralateral surgery is rarely required to achieve symmetry. Volume replacement reconstruction techniques are being employed more frequently as the indications for breast conservation therapy are extended to include larger T2 and T3 breast tumors, including those treated with adjuvant chemotherapy or radiation.[7] Unfortunately, some patients present requesting reconstruction for an unforeseen cosmetic defect after completion of BCT and radiation. These patients also benefit from autologous tissue transfer for volume replacement. This chapter focuses on the latissimus dorsi (LD) flap, the most commonly used autologous tissue in volume replacement reconstruction of the partial mastectomy defect following breast conserving surgery.

The LD flap was first described by Tansini in 1897. Evolving over the past century, this flap has been used reliably to cover soft tissue defects as a free or pedicle-based myocutaneous or myofascial flap.[8] The harvesting technique, which involves a large dorsal skin incision for flap elevation, has remained essentially the same since its initial introduction for soft tissue coverage of anterior chest wall defects.[9] The conventional technique, although clearly efficacious, results in a large oblique back scar that can be troubling to a woman concerned with cosmesis. In an era of oncoplastic breast resection and in a quest to combat unwanted scarring, the LD flap may also be harvested through an endoscopic approach.

The use of endoscopes to assist in partial mastectomy defect reconstruction has been effectively used at our institution since 1994. The endoscopic assisted reconstruction with latissimus dorsi (EARLi) flap technique, originally performed by the senior author after BCT, uses a much smaller incision (**Fig. 8.1**) than the open technique and is performed with the use of modified instruments used in endoscopic cholecystectomy surgery (**Fig. 8.2**). Less traumatic tissue dissection in conjunction with smaller surgical incisions have enabled many patients to benefit from reduced postoperative pain, expedited recovery, and improved cosmesis.[10] By comparison with other surgical disciplines, plastic surgery has been slower to adopt minimally invasive techniques, in part due to the limited surgical apertures, confined optical cavities, and difficult anatomical exposures required in many of the reconstructive procedures.[11] Improvement in general endoscopy in recent years and the addition of tumescent fluid has resulted in striking new advances in the technique of endoscopic latissimus harvest.[12]

BCT and reconstruction with the LD flap is an oncologically safe treatment for patients with early-stage breast cancer and those with larger T2 and T3 breast cancers.[7] At our institution, if a skin paddle is not necessary then we prefer the EARLi flap technique to achieve a favorable cosmetic outcome with little scarring. Because of the small incision and limited soft tissue dissection, postoperative pain is reduced and recovery time is diminished. Whether harvested through an open or endoscopic approach, the principal goals of the LD flap for reconstruction of partial mastectomy defects are to replace excised tissue volume and prevent breast deformity. In addition, breast size and contour are maintained, and scar tissue contracture is minimized.

Indications and contraindications

Significant volume loss after BCT surgery can result in a partial mastectomy defect requiring reconstruction with volume displacement or volume replacement oncoplastic techniques. Certain patients can be anticipated to have poor aesthetic outcomes after BCT. Recognizing patient and treatment-related risk factors at the time of consultation can optimize surgical planning and reconstructive options. Patient risk factors include large tumor size, patients with small breast to tumor ratios and tumor position, specifically superior medial tumors, and inferior lateral tumors.[13] Although there is a trend toward managing larger breast tumors with BCT, one of the major limi-

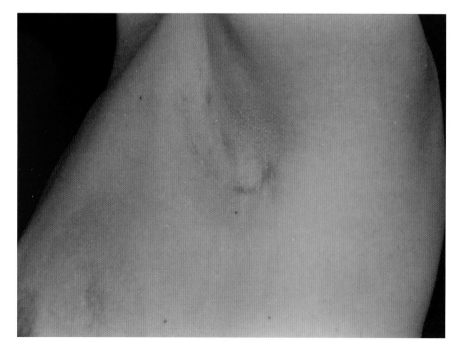

Figure 8.1 Left axillary scar after endoscopic LD harvest. The incision is made just large enough to accommodate the surgeon's hand and is well hidden in the axilla.

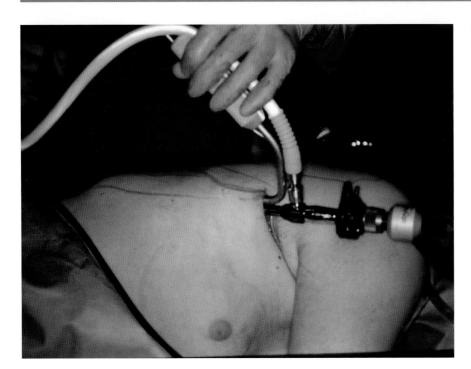

Figure 8.2 Endoscope insertion through the axillary incision.

tations is the ability to perform a large enough resection without compromising the cosmetic result. If anticipated breast volume excised is greater than 10–20%, then reconstruction should be planned.[3] Excising this amount of tissue in a small to medium-breasted woman without ptosis precludes the use of volume displacement techniques, whereas an LD flap reconstruction will provide optimal contour and shape. Treatment-related risk factors may include patients presenting with breast deformity following multiple re-excisions for positive margins or following the radiation phase of BCT.[13] Delayed reconstruction after radiation treatment is best managed with volume replacement using autologous tissue. In this situation, the LD flap will not only provide non-irradiated supple skin but also additional blood supply for adequate wound healing in an irradiated operative field.[14]

Partial mastectomy defects reconstructed with volume displacement techniques will usually require a contralateral breast symmetry procedure. Patients who are not amenable to surgery on the contralateral breast are good candidates for breast volume replacement techniques. This indication for an LD flap achieves a good breast contour and shape while maintaining volume to match the symmetry of the opposite breast.

The LD flap is optimal for defects in the upper outer quadrant, the site of occurrence for approximately 75% of breast cancers. This type of reconstruction is least suited for breast defects in the lower inner quadrant, where less than 6% of breast cancers reside. A large cavity in the lower inner quadrant cannot be adequately filled with a pedicled LD flap.

Due to the reliable and robust blood supply of the flap, patients with comorbidities that would preclude transfer of other autologous tissues are considered safe candidates for pedicled latissimus dorsi reconstruction. We have used this flap safely in patients with diabetes, smokers and in obese patients. General contraindications to oncoplastic reconstruction with volume replacement techniques include patients with T4 tumors, multicentric disease, extensive malignant mammographic microcalcifications, inflammatory carcinoma and when clear margins cannot be assured without performing a mastectomy.[15] The specific contraindications for an EARLi flap are essentially the same as those for a traditional LD flap. The exception occurs more in the event of delayed reconstruction. Patients presenting with radiation-induced deformities or other etiologies requiring need of a skin paddle for reconstruction are not candidates for the EARLi flap. Lack of latissimus musculature to adequately fill the oncologic resection defect would compromise breast shape and fail to achieve aesthetically pleasing cosmesis. This may be overcome with use of an implant or a contralateral breast-reducing procedure if the patient is amenable. Pedicle compromise is also a contraindication to the LD flap. A previous thoracotomy or axillary incision should raise the concern of an injured or ligated pedicle. The LD can survive on flow through the serratus branches if the thoracodorsal is the only vessel injured, but this would have to be carefully evaluated at the time of surgery. Other options for reconstruction would have to be discussed at the time of initial consultation in anticipation of previous injury to both arterial supplies.

Because the LD muscle is transferred, muscle function may be compromised, but functional deficits are only seen with specific activities. This flap would have relative contraindications in women active in sports requiring extreme upper body strength, such as mountain climbers, rowers and competitive swimmers, because muscle weakness can be seen in these patients.[16]

Preoperative history and considerations

Oncoplastic surgery is a new paradigm shift created in the evolution of multidisciplinary contributions to advancing breast cancer treatments. Conventionally, the breast surgeon ensured oncologic resection of the tumor and the patient was referred to a plastic surgeon for aesthetic breast reconstruction. Due to the new sub-specialty of oncoplastic surgery, oncologic principles and aesthetics are merging. There remains ambiguity as to the boundaries of breast surgeons and plastic surgeons when reconstructing a breast defect. Regardless, as the reconstructive surgeon, there are several underlying principles to understand and apply when initially evaluating a patient who is to receive BCT. To effectively care for these patients, the surgeon must be able to visualize the anticipated defect, all of its reconstructive options and be able to treat all potential postoperative complications.

Preoperative knowledge of the tumor location and size in comparison to the native breast volume is of high importance since volume displacement procedures are only suitable for patients with enough remaining healthy breast tissue to allow reconstruction of the breast. Discussing with patients their desires of having a symmetry procedure to the contralateral breast is necessary in the decision regarding reconstructive options. Volume replacement techniques such as the LD flap will be more suited to women who do not desire surgery to the opposite breast and who have large tumor to breast volume ratios. The location of the tumor plays a role in reconstructive options as medial lower quadrant defects in a patient with insufficient volume for breast displacement procedures will not be a good candidate for LD flap reconstruction and would be better served with autologous tissue from the abdomen.

Once volume replacement reconstruction is decided, patient history and desire will dictate whether LD reconstruction is chosen. Careful examination and past medical history will reveal any previous surgeries which may have compromised the vascular supply to the flap. Thoracotomy or axillary scars may preclude use of the thoracodorsal pedicle. Patients should be warned of the large donor site scar and given the option of an endoscopic approach. In the event of recurrence and need for a mastectomy, the option of an ipsilateral pedicled LD flap breast reconstruction will no longer be possible. In patients who desire autologous reconstruction, evaluation of the abdominal tissues is necessary, so that in the event of recurrence and completion mastectomy they may be easily reconstructed with TRAM flaps.[17]

A patient may present for consultation after completion of breast conservation therapy with a significant breast deformity. This type of secondary reconstruction for radiated partial mastectomy deformities can be more difficult to correct. The breast resection not only creates loss of volume, but the radiation results in soft tissue scarring and contracture which may distort the nipple–areola complex. These patients will often need a skin paddle in addition to soft tissues for volume replacement and therefore will not qualify for an endoscopic approach. It is not advisable to offer these patients delayed breast displacement techniques as the complication rate averages 50% due to decreased healing properties of the irradiated local tissues.[14]

Timing of the partial mastectomy defect reconstruction using the LD flap is a critical component to success with this technique. The reconstruction is performed only after wide local excision and confirmation of final pathology reports. It should not be used simultaneously at the time of initial tumor resection before final margins are confirmed. With immediate reconstruction it is difficult to locate the position of a positive tumor margin. If the final pathology is back, the procedure can be performed early in the postoperative period, as early as 3 days after oncologic resection. However, it may also be performed as a delayed–immediate reconstruction as long as 3 weeks after tumor resection to accommodate patient preference for timing of surgery. This approach will not sacrifice an important reconstructive modality if the breast and flap need to be removed to obtain adequate tumor margins.[17] While a short interval between lumpectomy and LD flap reconstruction is important, it is advantageous to carry out the flap prior to the formation of scar contracture in order to obviate the need for a skin paddle to release contracted skin.

Reconstruction with an LD flap does not affect postoperative cancer surveillance,[18] which is important since some studies have found 2-to 3-year local recurrence rates to be as high as 13–15% when using an LD flap for volume replacement.[14,17] This number seems high when compared to the reported 8–22% 18-year recurrence rates following traditional lumpectomy techniques.[19] Our institution-based local recurrence rates correlate more with the 6% rates seen in the literature following displacement oncoplastic techniques.[14] We believe that local recurrence rates are institution based due to different resection techniques and patient selection variations. Many of the patients receiving LD flap volume replacement have larger tumors and may be better served with a mastectomy and reconstruction. If an LD reconstruction is chosen, then higher chances of local recurrence will need to be discussed with the patients. To reduce the rate, breast tumor resection is best treated with oncoplastic techniques rather than by simple lumpectomy. If larger volumes are removed, such as in the case of a partial mastectomy or quadrantectomy, then wider margins will naturally be obtained, resulting in lower rates of local recurrence. Invariably, local recurrences will continue to occur throughout the follow-up period, so close surveillance is warranted. Recurrence may present as a palpable nodule that can be easily biopsied for pathologic review. For non-palpable recurrences, women treated with LD flap reconstruction after BCT have mammographic findings that are predictable. The most common radiographic appearances are relative radiolucency in the central portion of the flap due to fibrofatty degeneration, with or without density from muscle fibers at the periphery of the transferred LD.[18]

Operative approach

Relevant anatomy

The LD is a large flat muscle arising from the posterior iliac crest, the caudal six thoracic vertebrae and the lumbosacral spinous processes. It inserts on the lesser tubercle and intertubercular groove of the humerus, allowing extension, adduction and medial rotation of the shoulder. The superior edge of the LD covers the tip of the scapula and fuses with a portion of the teres major laterally. Medially, the superior edge of the LD is covered by the trapezius muscle. The LD overlies and is adherent to the serratus anterior, fibers of the external oblique muscle, and the lower four ribs. The thick fibrous aponeurosis between the LD and the serratus is surgically important at the inferior edge of the serratus muscle at approximately the 10th rib. Knowledge of this anatomy is important when dissecting beneath the LD to avoid accidental elevation of the serratus.

The LD muscle is supplied by one dominant pedicle, the thoracodorsal artery, as well as segmental intercostals and lumbar perforators which penetrate the undersurface of the muscle near the posterior midline. Before entering the LD muscle, the thoracodorsal artery gives off one or two branches to the serratus anterior. Once inside the LD muscle the artery branches, forming a robust vascular network. Perforators supplying the skin are abundant, allowing creativity in design of a skin paddle if necessary. The neural innervation of the LD muscle is supplied by the thoracodorsal nerve, which accompanies the path of its co-named artery and vein.

Open latissimus dorsi flap

Preoperative markings should be made prior to positioning the patient on the operating room table. Ideally, the patient is marked in an upright standing or seated position. If a skin island is needed, then it is drawn overlying the LD. If extra volume is needed but the patient has a sufficient skin envelope then a skin island may be harvested and de-epithelialized prior to inset. Although the island can be designed in any direction, it is best to consider orienting the scar along relaxed skin tension lines instead of trying to hide the scar in the bra line. Whether the patient requires a skin island or not, the scar from the open approach has been less conspicuous using this approach to incision placement. Assurance of skin closure without tension is performed by pinching the back skin and soft tissues together at the boundaries of the skin paddle markings.

After the induction of general anesthesia, the patient is placed in a lateral decubitus position, with the operative side up. A vacuum-molded pad or bean bag is placed beneath the patient in order to maintain position throughout the operation. The arm on the side of the defect is prepped into the operative field so it can be moved to allow optimal visualization during the procedure. The primary surgeon stands facing the patient's anterior chest, whereas the assistant stands facing the patient's back.

Tumescence fluid is minimally infused into the tissues at the planned skin incision sites to ensure local hemostasis. The scar created by the breast surgeon for wide local excision is opened first to fully appreciate the soft tissue defect. In the case of delayed reconstruction due to breast deformity after BCT with radiation, the scarred and contracted tissue is resected, thereby creating a defect. The width of the skin paddle necessary for delayed reconstruction of the partial mastectomy defect is dependent on the amount of skin that may be safely removed to allow closure of the back tissues. In the case of delayed immediate reconstruction with only deficiencies in parenchymal volume, the extent of distal LD liberation depends on the amount of tissue required to fill the breast defect. In either case, the quantity of transferred LD muscle should be tailored to provide an aesthetically contoured breast mound. The amount of additional subfascial fatty tissue incorporated onto the superficial aspect of the LD flap is gauged to appropriately augment the reconstruction of a large defect. Dissection begins from within the resection defect, creating a tunnel towards the axilla through which the flap will pass. If possible, the lateral margin of the LD muscle should be identified to allow for ease of passage after harvesting the flap.

Next, attention is turned to the back for flap elevation. The skin is incised sharply and dissection is continued down through the superficial fascia which clearly separates the fatty component of the back into two layers. The more superficial layer is responsible for maintaining back contour and must not be taken with the muscle, with the exception of cases necessitating a skin paddle, in which the superficial fascia in conjunction with the skin paddle is sacrificed as an island only. Importantly, if the superficial fat is inadvertently harvested with the muscle, the back skin flaps will be unreliable since their blood supply is partially dependent on perforators emanating from the fascia dividing the fatty tissue layers. The deeper, subfascial fatty tissue layer can be harvested attached to the LD muscle to create bulk if needed to fill the defect. If this layer is included with the flap, it should be preserved in its entirety and not just over a portion of the muscle. In this way, the back contour remains uniform. If the volume harvested is more than needed, excess fat can always be trimmed at the time of inset. The extent of dissection overlying the LD muscle is determined by evaluating the breast resection defect prior to harvest. If the entire muscle is needed, then dissection is carried out to the previously mentioned landmarks which delineate the muscle boundaries. Superiorly, the deep fatty tissue overlying the LD muscle is incised along the medial border until the obliquely oriented trapezius muscle is identified. Beneath this muscle, the superior edge of the LD can be easily located. By placing a finger beneath the LD and applying tension away from the chest wall, a plane can be easily entered. The superior attachments are released first extending laterally toward the axilla. Next the medial attachments are released, taking care to adequately cauterize or ligate the large paraspinal perforators. Next, the inferior and inferolateral attachments are released. As the dissection is carried out in a caudal to cranial direction along the anterior surface of the LD, care must be taken not to elevate the serratus muscle with the LD. Here, a thick fibrous attachment exists between the LD and the serratus which must be divided to remain in the appropriate sub-latissimus plane (**Fig. 8.3**). As dissection proceeds toward the muscle insertion, the pedicle will become apparent on the anterior surface of the latissimus. Once the neurovascular pedicle is identified and protected, the muscle insertion is completely divided. It is not necessary to divide the thoracodorsal nerve. The pivotal role of the LD flap is to restore volume; muscle atrophy, as a result of deinnervation, would be counterproductive. Dividing the muscle insertion eliminates dyskinetic pulling of the arm and breast, which can be problematic if the nerve is left intact and the insertion is not divided. The portion of the tunnel within the axilla may have to be extended to connect with the previously created tunnel from the resec-

tion defect. At this point the flap should be completely free of any other attachments and easily transposed through the tunnel and guided into the partial mastectomy defect. After the flap is adequately positioned to fill the breast defect, 3-0 Vicryl sutures are used to loosely tack the muscle in its final position. Two 7 mm Axiom Clot Stop drains are placed into the donor site on the back and one is placed into the breast. A local anesthetic catheter may be inserted into the axilla to assist with postoperative pain management. The donor site and breast incisions are each closed with interrupted 3-0 Vicryl deep sutures and running 4-0 Prolene subcuticular sutures. Typical operative time is less than 2 hours (**Figs 8.4** and **8.5**).

Endoscopic latissimus dorsi flap

Patient positioning on the operating room table is the same for both the endoscopic and open approaches. Tumescence fluid is also used in the endoscopic technique, but it is infused into the subcutaneous tissues overlying the LD muscle to facilitate not only local hemostasis but also atraumatic tissue plane dissection. Typical volumes of tumescent fluid are 500–1000 cm³, depending on the size of the patient. As with the open technique, the existing breast incision is opened and the extent of the soft tissue defect is appreciated. This allows time for the epinephrine in the tumescent fluid to take effect and also allows for estimation of the amount of LD needed to fill the defect. A curvilinear incision is then made in the axilla along the inferior hair line. The length of the incision is variable and is tailored to accommodate the size of the surgeon's hand. The typical incision length

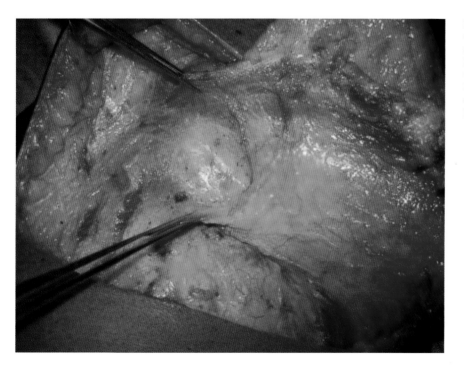

Figure 8.3 Anatomy of the LD and serratus during open LD harvest. The upper forceps are shown grasping the latissimus muscle and the lower forceps are shown grasping the serratus muscle. Note the thick fibrous attachment between these two muscles that must be divided to remain in the correct sub-latissimus plane.

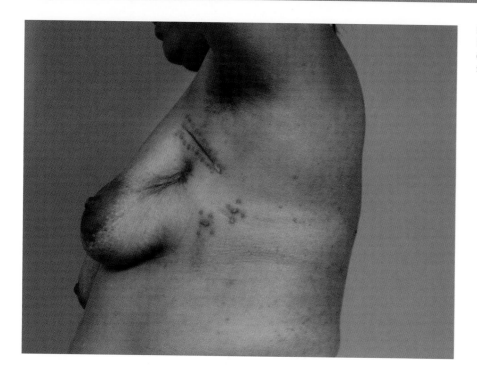

Figure 8.4 Preoperative view of a delayed lumpectomy defect with significant skin contracture and loss of volume, requiring both skin and soft tissue for adequate reconstruction.

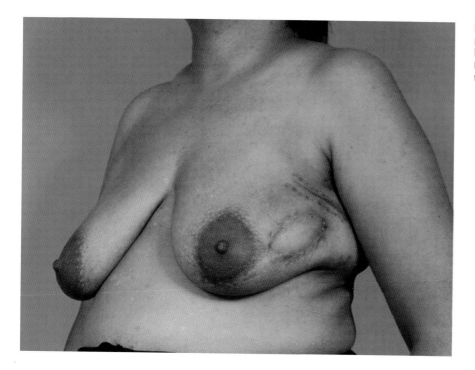

Figure 8.5 Postoperative view of the same patient. After excision of contracted skin, the lumpectomy defect is successfully replaced with LD flap and overlying skin paddle using an open technique.

is approximately 9 cm. In patients who have previously undergone transaxillary sentinel lymph node sampling, the incision incorporates the existing scar line. If the previous breast incision is high in the upper outer quadrant, it may also be used for the LD dissection.

Initial dissection is focused on identification of the thoracodorsal pedicle, which is located along the lateral edge of the LD muscle. Once the thoracodorsal pedicle is unequivocally identified, arterial tributaries supplying the serratus anterior must be clip-ligated and divided. The serratus branch must be ligated to allow full LD elevation without risk of avulsion. Because of the high axillary incision the thoracodorsal pedicle may be mistaken for the serratus branch, so care must be exercised at this point.

The deep surface of the LD muscle is then elevated off the chest wall using a combination of monopolar electrocautery with blunt and sharp dissection. The surgeon's hand is inserted to assist with blunt dissection and to ensure the proper plane of dissection by palpating the scapula below the plane of dissection. It is easy to slip below deep to the scapula. This is the wrong plane and should be avoided. A retractor with an endoscope, or a lighted retractor, is then introduced into the operative field and utilized to facilitate mobilization of the LD from its myofascial attachments. Lumbar perforators may be visualized and clipped or cauterized using endoscopic guidance at this point. The perforators may also be bluntly avulsed. They do not bleed due to the tumescent fluid. They will be cauterized at the conclusion of the procedure. After completing the deep dissection plane, sharp dissection with scissors is used to free the anterior and posterior border of the muscle. Initially, this is done via direct vision, then endoscopic visualization is used, followed by 'blind' pushing of the scissors to get maximal length of the muscle. The scissors used are typically long Metzenbaum's with some use of the endoscopic 10 mm scissors. The next step is to dissect the superficial surface. Initially, this is done directly on top of the muscle. This tissue will end up in the axilla so extra bulk is not needed. After 5–6 cm on the muscle the plane of dissection transitions to just below the fascia separating the two fatty layers overlying the LD. This adds a layer of fat to the muscle, increasing the bulk and allowing larger defects to be adequately filled. The procedure for this dissection is the same as freeing the edges, first direct vision, then some endoscopic work, and finally blind or externally visualized dissection with progressively longer Metzenbaum's and endoscopic scissors.

At this point in the procedure, the LD is left adherent to only its distal origin along the thoracolumbar vertebral column and posterior iliac crest, and its insertion on the humerus. The distal extent of the muscular flap is sharply divided using tactile guidance and endoscopic scissors. The division of the distal muscular origin is the most challenging part of the procedure. The senior author has tried many methods and has found sharp division with tactile guidance to be the most efficient. Tactile guidance refers to the technique whereby the surgeon inserts one hand into the incision and grips the distal muscle between the thumb and fingers and then cuts just beyond the finger tips with endoscopic scissors. The surgeon's hand provides both guidance and traction and greatly facilitates this portion of the procedure. It is at this point that many surgeons may want to hesitate in proceeding with sharp division of muscle due to concerns over bleeding. However, active bleeding is not a problem with this or any other part of the procedure due to the hemostatic effect of the epinephrine in the tumescent fluid instilled at the beginning of the procedure. After distal division is complete, the muscle is delivered through the axillary incision (**Fig. 8.6**).

The muscle flap is carefully examined and hemostasis is achieved with the aid of bipolar electrocautery. Special attention is given to identify the number and location of lumbar and intercostal perforators severed during mobilization of the LD flap as this will play a role in final hemostasis prior to closure. These vessels usually are not actively bleeding, due to the tumescent fluid, but they can be seen. The insertion of the muscle into the humerus is completely divided using monopolar electrocautery, which allows for further anterior arc rotation to reach defects in a more medial location. This also limits pulling on the arm and breast with subsequent muscle flexion. After complete mobilization of the LD, the flap is tethered

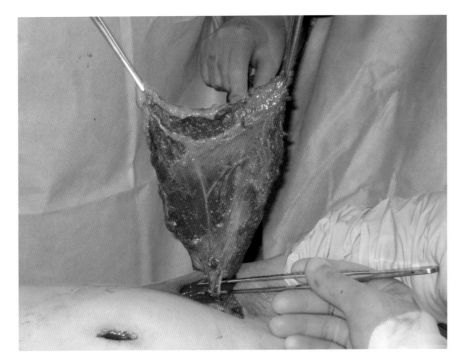

Figure 8.6 LD muscle flap delivered into the axillary incision.

only by its neurovascular pedicle. As with the open approach, the thoracodorsal nerve is not divided. Not only is there concern for muscle atrophy, but the innervated muscle may now serve as a monitoring modality for the completely buried flap. By asking the patient to push their elbow into the surgeon's hand, the LD contracts, which may be palpated at the breast surgical site. Creation of a subcutaneous tunnel proceeds from the axillary incision into the breast defect. The muscle is then passed through the tunnel and guided into the breast defect through the existing breast resection site. After the flap is adequately positioned to fill the breast defect, 3-0 Vicryl sutures are used to loosely tack the muscle in its final position.

Attention is now turned to the donor site. This is the portion of the operation that truly depends on the endoscope. Using the endoscope, perforators are identified and coagulated along the posterior midline. Curved, insulated endoscopic grasping forceps are used to coagulate the most posterior vessels. The number and location of bleeding sites should correspond to perforators identified on the muscle during flap hemostasis. It is rarely necessary to coagulate any vessels in the cut edge of the muscle. Generally, only lumbar and intercostal vessels are coagulated. Two 7 mm Axiom Clot Stop drains are placed into the donor site on the back and one is placed into the breast. A local anesthetic catheter may be inserted into the axilla to assist with postoperative pain management. The axillary and breast incisions are each closed with interrupted 3-0 Vicryl deep sutures and running 4-0 Prolene subcuticular sutures. Typical operative time is between 2 and 3 hours (**Figs 8.7–8.10**).

Optimizing outcomes

- Volume restoration with autologous tissue is preferred when the tumor size in relation to the breast size is large enough to prohibit cosmetically acceptable results using local glandular rearrangement techniques. In general, if more than 20% of the breast volume is excised, then an LD flap is an excellent choice for volume replacement, especially if the patient is not amenable to a contralateral breast symmetry procedure.
- EARLi flap: infuse tumescent fluid and use sharp division of the distal LD muscular origin along with tactile guidance to make the procedure significantly less complicated. Bleeding is not a problem due to tumescent fluid and endoscopic hemostasis evaluation.
- Delayed–immediate reconstruction is the safest way to ensure negative surgical margins and not waste a valuable reconstructive option in the event of positive pathology at the resection boundaries.

Complications and side effects

The LD flap reconstruction has proven to be a reliable and safe procedure. With its robust blood supply, this flap infrequently suffers significant necrosis unless the pedicle is inadvertently injured during the harvest or in the case of an axillary dissection. Postoperative complications after endoscopically assisted and open LD flap breast reconstruction are comparable. The most common

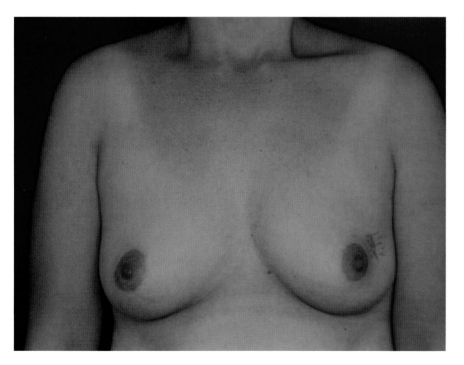

Figure 8.7 Preoperative view of a left lumpectomy defect.

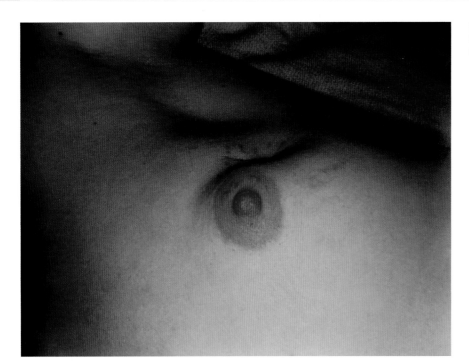

Figure 8.8 Close-up view of the same patient in a lateral decubitus position before re-excision, showing extent of the defect.

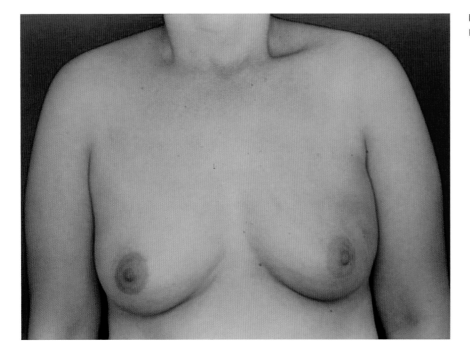

Figure 8.9 Postoperative view of the same patient after left EARLi flap reconstruction.

complication is donor site seromas, which can usually be managed by percutaneous office aspiration. There are no significant differences in donor site hematomas or seromas when comparing the endoscopically assisted and traditional harvest techniques. EARLi flaps tend to have less pain and allow for early upper extremity movement and overall improved cosmesis over the open approach.[20] Delayed wound healing and scar widening can occur with the open technique and is a disadvantage when compared to the endoscopic harvest. Depressed back contour can occur with either approach if fat is taken superficial to the fascia. Shoulder complications, including temporary stiffness and weakness, can present immediately after surgery. Prolonged arm abduction during the muscle harvest can be a contributing factor. If symptoms persist after the acute phase of surgery, physical therapy should be initiated.

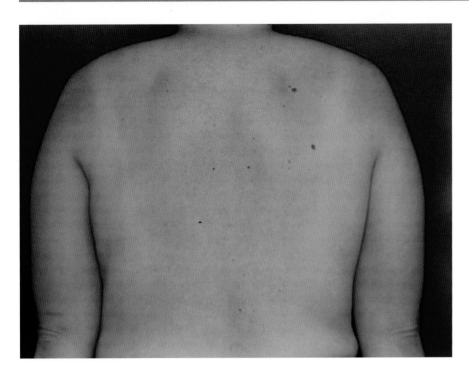

Figure 8.10 Posterior postoperative view of the same patient, illustrating minimal back deformity after LD harvest. Lack of a large back scar is cosmetically appealing.

Postoperative care

The surgical site is dressed with loosely applied bandages which are removed after approximately 24 hours. The postoperative hospital course is typically 24–48 hours and patients are encouraged to ambulate immediately. Typical suction drains are kept in place until the output is less than 30 cm^3 in a 24-hour period. A more conservative approach is often used to manage the back donor site drains secondary to high risk of postoperative seroma formation. Therefore, it is not unusual to have suction drains in place for 3–4 weeks after surgery. Daily living activities, including hair combing and teeth brushing, are encouraged immediately. Avoiding certain activities that may cause the LD to contract, such as pushing up off the bed with the affected arm, are discouraged initially. More strenuous physical activity, including lifting, can be resumed at 4–6 weeks. This time frame is a general guide-line. Some patients will complain of a stiff shoulder early in the postoperative course. These patients will need to start more strenuous range of motion exercises or physical therapy earlier than anticipated.

Conclusion

Oncoplastic breast surgery has expanded the indications of breast conservation therapy. Through the use of volume replacement techniques, specifically the latissimus dorsi muscle flap, extensive resections that satisfy oncologic principles and reconstruction to achieve good cosmesis can now be simultaneously obtained. Through a transaxillary approach, endoscopic breast reconstruction using the EARLi technique has enabled women to achieve an aesthetically pleasing result with minimal scarring and fast recovery.

References

1. Fisher B, Anderson S, Redmond CK, et al. Reanalysis and results after 12 years of follow-up in a randomized clinical trial comparing total mastectomy with lumpectomy with or without irradiation in the treatment of breast cancer. N Engl J Med 1995; 333(22):1456–1461.
2. Zoetmulder FA, Borger JH, Rutgers EJ, et al. Breast conserving therapy in patients with relatively large (T2, T3) breast cancers by preoperative irradiation and myocutaneous LD flap reconstruction: a new technique in breast conservation. Eur J Cancer 1993; 29A(7):957–961.
3. Cochrane RA, Valasiadou P, Wilson AR, et al. Cosmesis and satisfaction after breast-conserving surgery correlates with the percentage of breast volume excised. Br J Surg 2003; 90(12):1505–1509.
4. Giacalone PL, Roger P, Dubon O, et al. Comparative study of the accuracy of breast resection in oncoplastic surgery and quadrantectomy in breast cancer. Ann Surg Oncol 2007; 14(2):605–614.
5. Kerlikowske K, Molinaro A, Cha I, et al. Characteristics associated with recurrence among women with ductal carcinoma in situ treated by lumpectomy. J Natl Cancer Inst 2003; 95(22):1692–1702.
6. Bulstrode NW, Shrotria S. Prediction of cosmetic outcome following conservative breast surgery using breast volume measurements. Breast 2001; 10(2):124–126.
7. Woerdeman LA, Haje JJ, Thio EA, et al. Breast-conserving therapy in patients with a relatively large (T2 or T3) breast cancer: long-term local control and cosmetic outcome of a feasibility study. Plast Reconstr Surg 2004; 113(6):1607–1616.
8. Maxwell GP. Iginio Tansini and the origin of the latissimus dorsi

musculocutaneous flap. Plast Reconstr Surg 1980; 65(5):686–692.

9. Bostwick J 3rd, Vasconez LO, Jurkiewicz MJ. Breast reconstruction after a radical mastectomy. Plast Reconstr Surg 1978; 61(5):682–693.

10. Cho BC, Lee JH, Ramasastry SS, et al. Free latissimus dorsi muscle transfer using an endoscopic technique. Ann Plast Surg 1997; 38(6):586–593.

11. Vasconez LO, Core GB, Oslin B. Endoscopy in plastic surgery: an overview. Clin Plast Surg 1995; 22(4):585–589.

12. Fine NA, Orgill DP, Pribaz JJ. Early clinical experience in endoscopic-assisted muscle flap harvest. Ann Plast Surg 1994; 33(5):465–469; discussion 469–472.

13. Waljee JF, Hu ES, Newman LA, et al. Predictors of breast asymmetry after breast-conserving operation for breast cancer. J Am Coll Surg 2008; 206(2):274–280.

14. Kronowitz SJ, Feledy JA, Hunt KK, et al. Determining the optimal approach to breast reconstruction after partial mastectomy. Plast Reconstr Surg 2006; 117(1):1–11; discussion 12–14.

15. Baildam A, Bishop H, Boland G, et al. Oncoplastic breast surgery: a guide to good practice. Eur J Surg Oncol 2007; 33(Suppl 1):S1–23.

16. Fraulin FO, Louie G, Zorrilla L, et al. Functional evaluation of the shoulder following latissimus dorsi muscle transfer. Ann Plast Surg 1995; 35(4):349–355.

17. Losken A, Schaeffer TG, Carlson GW, et al. Immediate endoscopic latissimus dorsi flap: risk or benefit in reconstructing partial mastectomy defects. Ann Plast Surg 2004; 53(1): 1–5.

18. Monticciolo DL, Ross D, Bostwick J 3rd, et al. Autologous breast reconstruction with endoscopic latissimus dorsi musculosubcutaneous flaps in patients choosing breast-conserving therapy: mammographic appearance. Am J Roentgenol 1996; 167(2):385–389.

19. Poggi MM, Danforth DN, Sciuto LC, et al. Eighteen-year results in the treatment of early breast carcinoma with mastectomy versus breast conservation therapy: the National Cancer Institute Randomized Trial. Cancer 2003; 98(4):697–702.

20. Lin CH, Wei FC, Levin LS, et al. Donor-site morbidity comparison between endoscopically assisted and traditional harvest of free latissimus dorsi muscle flap. Plast Reconstr Surg 1999; 104(4):1070–1077; quiz 1078.

CHAPTER 9

Repair of the Partial Mastectomy Defect with Delayed Free Tissue Transfer

Moustapha Hamdi • Jonathan Cheng

Introduction

Breast conservation therapy (BCT) may be considered a mainstay therapy for early-stage breast cancer[1] and an oncological equivalent to mastectomy in selected cases.[2,3] As reviewed elsewhere in this text, BCT comprises partial breast resection, lymph node dissection, and whole breast irradiation. Specifically, for Stage I and II breast cancer, no significant difference was found in overall or disease-free survival between BCT and mastectomy after follow-up times of up to 20 years.[2–10] The most important difference which has been identified between BCT and mastectomy is a significantly higher rate of local recurrence after BCT. This was found in only two of the six existing randomized controlled trials,[7–9] and the differences are of questionable relevance to current practice given the lack of microscopic margin control in those two trials.[11]

Although the oncologic outcome is well defined, the ultimate aesthetic outcome after BCT remains highly variable. Conventional reports in the radiation oncology literature indicate unsatisfactory appearance in 10–31% of patients following BCT at late reporting by patients or radiation oncologists.[12–14] In fact, 50% of post-BCT aesthetic results were only considered to be fair or poor when assessed by a plastic surgeon at 34 months median follow-up.[15]

Specific conditions which lead to poor aesthetic outcomes following BCT have been described. In absolute terms, if cancer removal requires excision of more than 25% of the breast parenchyma or a large amount of skin, a poor aesthetic outcome can be anticipated.[16] In relative terms, the size of the tumor excision must be compared to the size of the affected breast in order to estimate the final aesthetic impact. Three specific scenarios have been identified as unfavorable: (1) a large excision in a very large breast; (2) a medium excision in a small breast; and (3) a large excision in a small or medium breast.[16] To summarize, the larger the breast, the more easily it accommodates larger resections up to a certain size; small to medium breasts are far less tolerant of increasing resection sizes than large breasts.

Our preference is to perform immediate reconstruction for the scenarios described above. Clinical outcomes[15,17,18] and expert impressions[16,19–23] support this approach. These sources suggest that post-BCT breast contour deformity develops primarily from an inappropriate surgical defect and secondarily from the injury and fibrosis induced by radiotherapy. In other words, radiotherapy tends to 'exaggerate' the surgically created deformity, but the aesthetic impact of BCT can be minimized by performing oncoplastic or reconstructive surgery to fill the unfavorable resection cavity with local or distant tissues prior to administering radiation.[21] Immediate reconstruction has definite advantages over delayed reconstruction, as lower complication rates and substantially more straightforward corrections can be expected because the surgical field has not received prior irradiation with its widespread implications for tissue injury and scarring.[23-25]

If immediate reconstruction is not performed in cases with unfavorable resection defects, significant breast deformities will likely manifest following completion of the BCT regimen. These deformities have been stratified by two major competing schemas. Berrino and colleagues were the first to classify post-BCT deformities, by identifying the morphology of the deformity and then referencing this to select a technique for correction.[26] They described the following deformity types: (I) displacement of the nipple–areolar complex; (II) localized deficiency of parenchyma and/or skin; (III) generalized breast contracture with no localized defects; (IV) severe damage with heavily scarred parenchyma and skin. Clough et al have altered this classification by reordering and combining groups, emphasizing reconstructive choices, and including comparison with the opposite breast.[22] Their three types are: (I) deformity of the affected breast with no contour defects and leading to asymmetry with the contralateral breast; (II) deformity requiring delayed partial reconstruction; (III) severe deformity requiring mastectomy and whole breast reconstruction. In clinical application, these classifications help to clarify the deformities which typically result when BCT is performed under suboptimal conditions. The classification schema also guides us in reconstruction by emphasis on identifying what is missing or disordered and on seeking a reasonable match between the two breasts.

When these post-BCT deformities occur, delayed partial breast reconstruction must be considered. We consider these cases to be difficult and fraught with potential problems on three separate fronts. First, these patients often present to us with ongoing disappointment about their breast appearance following BCT, and with higher cosmetic expectations than when they were in the primary cancer treatment phase. Second, breasts previously treated with BCT present limited options[23,27] for reconstruction due to reduced breast volume, scarring, distorted anatomy, and disturbed vascularity. Third, post-radiation changes must be approached with caution, as correction is technically difficult and results and complications are highly unpredictable.[24] Studies have estimated the complication rate to be as high as 50%[25] and the final aesthetic result to be poor[18,22] when extensive tissue rearrangement is performed in the previously irradiated breast. Owing to these serious concerns, we limit post-BCT reconstruction to contralateral symmetry procedures, local flaps, or scar revisions requiring minimal dissection of the affected breast, and importing of distant tissues, pedicled or free, to correct the skin and/or parenchymal deficiencies.

Indications and contraindications

Our algorithm for recruiting distant tissues for partial breast reconstruction is to turn first to pedicled flaps and then to free flaps if pedicled flaps are insufficient or unavailable. Conventional pedicled flap options include the latissimus dorsi (LD) muscle or myocutaneous flap and the transverse rectus abdominis myocutaneous (TRAM) flap. These have been shown to be perfectly suitable for breast reconstruction following irradiation, with the accepted caveats of higher complication rates and poorer aesthetic results.[24] The muscular component of the flaps is transferred in a denervated state, so any attempt to utilize muscle for parenchymal replacement must include substantial overcorrection to account for future denervation atrophy.[18,27] Despite good results with the TRAM flap, we strongly discourage its use for partial breast reconstruction due to concern that this tissue may be needed in the future for reconstruction after completion mastectomy for local breast cancer recurrence, or after primary mastectomy for cancer of the contralateral breast.[16,23,28,29] With the development of pedicled perforator flaps for partial breast reconstruction, more options and potentially lower donor site morbidity through muscle sparing are now available when a large amount of tissue is needed.[23,30,31] A particular anatomical limitation to the use of pedicled flaps for partial breast reconstruction must be noted. Laterally based pedicled flaps (i.e., LD, lateral intercostal artery perforator, thoracodorsal artery perforator, lateral thoracic) generally are not suitable for reconstruction of large defects of the medial breast quadrants due to insufficient reach. Although this is a recognized limitation, it is only acknowledged in a few reports on this topic.[23,25,27]

The TRAM is the only pedicled flap which reaches the medial breast quadrants easily.[32] Its use for partial breast reconstruction, however, generally must be discouraged because this eliminates the use of the abdominal wall flap for a local recurrence or a new tumor in the contralateral breast as discussed in the preceding paragraph.

In the experience of the senior author, indications are real but limited for delayed free flap reconstruction of partial mastectomy defects:

- for severe breast deformity (Clough Grade III) when non-abdominal pedicled flaps are inadequate or unavailable;
- for large breast deformity (Clough Grade II) in the medial quadrants;
- in conjunction with completion mastectomy for difficult tumor control or major glandular fibrosis post-irradiation (Berrino Grade IV);
- as part of treatment consisting of contralateral mastectomy (therapeutic or prophylactic) and correction of ipsilateral post-BCT deformity;
- with aesthetic abdominoplasty procedure in a patient with long-term follow-up and no further risk of recurrence or developing a new breast cancer.

Surgical technique

Preoperative assessment

The principles of using free tissue transfer for post-BCT deformity are summarized in **Table 9.1**. Thorough preoperative consultation is essential in order to explain the surgical plan, expected results, and potential high complication rate due to the post-radiotherapy status. Furthermore, every candidate for this technique should undergo a complete examination and check-up by the oncology team before considering an attempt at surgical correction. This examination must be comprehensive and should encompass the entire body, including the breasts. The author requests additional magnetic resonance imaging when there is any doubt in the interpretation of the preoperative mammogram or ultrasound examinations.

In our patients, preoperative radiological exams are routinely obtained for flap perforator mapping and recipient vessel evaluation. Color duplex examination gives valuable information about the intraluminal flow in both arteries and veins.[33] More recently, the multi-detector CT (MDCT) has been introduced into our preoperative assessment.[34] MDCT provides more accurate information about the location and diameter of perforators and vessels in general, but provides much less information about the veins due to technical limitations in obtaining venous-phase data.

Free flap selection

Flap planning should account for what is missing from the breast skin and parenchyma, but also should consider the reduced elasticity in the residual breast tissue. In a free flap reconstruction, an ample and adequate skin paddle should be available with proper planning. In our flap plethora, we consider perforator flaps to be the gold standard for reconstruction because of their low donor site morbidity.

Our first choice is the deep inferior epigastric artery perforator (DIEP) flap, because it provides an ample amount of soft tissue with good color and consistency match.[35–38] The superficial inferior epigastric artery (SIEA)

flap is a good alternative to the DIEP flap whenever the direct cutaneous SIE vessels are available and suitable in diameter to perform microanastomoses.[39,40,41] Alternative flaps include the superior gluteal artery perforator (SGAP) and the inferior gluteal artery perforator (IGAP) flaps, which may be considered for post-BCT reconstruction. However, in cases of bilateral free flap breast reconstruction, simultaneous bilateral SGAP or IGAP reconstruction is time consuming due to multiple patient repositionings. In our institute, bilateral gluteal flap surgery is usually performed in two stages with a 3- to 6-month interval between stages. The transverse myocutaneous gracilis (TMG) flap has become a valuable alternative to the gluteal perforator flaps, for bilateral reconstruction cases in particular, due to easy access to both donor sites without need for repositioning.[42–44]

Surgical technique

During surgery, all damaged skin, scar, and fibrotic tissue are excised. Frozen section examination can be requested if recurrence is suspected within the excised tissue. A completion subcutaneous mastectomy is usually performed: thicker skin flaps are developed, with preservation of internal mammary perforators to the medial breast tissues. This maximizes vascularity and thereby minimizes ischemic slough of the previously irradiated skin. We believe that by performing a completion subcutaneous mastectomy a significant reduction in the cancer recurrence rate and a more complete release of the post-irradiation parenchymal fibrosis can be achieved.

The recipient vessels should be carefully prepared if irradiation was given specifically to the selected region. We prefer the internal mammary vessels, because these vessels usually have less damage post BCT when compared to the thoracodorsal vessels (**Fig. 9.1**). In addition, sparing the thoracodorsal vessels allows future use of a pedicled TDAP or LD flap for breast salvage in the case of free flap failure or cancer recurrence.

DIEP flap

The technique of DIEP flap harvest requires several steps and close attention to detail. The location of the perforator vessels can be determined preoperatively using computed tomographic angiography. The outline of the flap is delineated on the lower anterior abdominal wall (**Fig. 9.2**). The superior and inferior margins of the flap are incised and the elevation of the flap proceeds in the lateral to medial direction. At this point, careful attention is given toward the location and identification of the dominant perforator or perforators. Once the perforator is isolated, the dissection is continued by incising the anterior rectus sheath and carefully releasing all fascial attachments to the perforator (**Fig. 9.3**). The dissection is continued, dividing all small branches that emanate from the perforator and the inferior epigastric artery and vein. The perforator flap is ultimately elevated until its sole attachment is via the common source vessel (**Fig. 9.4**). The

Table 9.1 Surgical principles

Careful planning of the flap and the recipient vessels
Radiological assessment of the vessels
Excision of damaged tissue – release of scar – re-creation of defect
Careful preparation of the internal mammary vessels
Free flap options – DIEP, SIEA, TRAM, TMG
Consideration of muscle sacrifice (overcorrection, atrophy, functional impairment)
Improvement of shaping (based on aesthetic subunits)
Surveillance for cancer

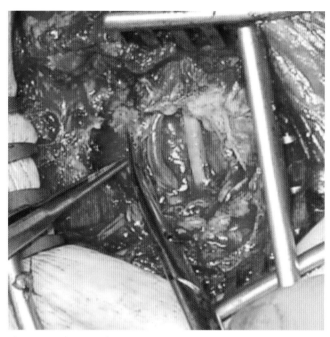

Figure 9.1 The internal mammary artery and vein are depicted. As recipient vessels, these are preferred because they are relatively easy to expose, and high flow, and allow for optimal flap insetting.

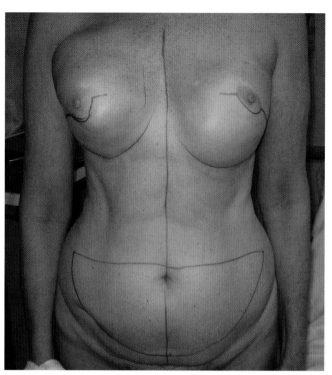

Figure 9.2 The outline for the abdominal based flaps is usually based on the anterior superior iliac spine as the lateral extension. The dominant perforators are usually located in the periumbilical area, so this portion of the flap is important to include. The superior extent of the flap is usually just above the umbilicus and the inferior extension of the flap is based on the excursion of the supraumbilical tissues.

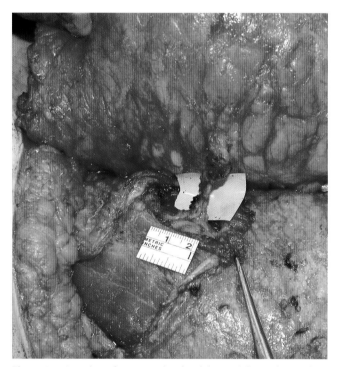

Figure 9.3 A single perforator is isolated and depicted during the initial portion of the perforator dissection.

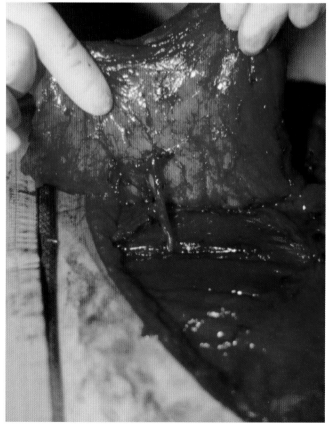

Figure 9.4 The DIEAP flap is elevated and maintained on a single pedicle. Adequate vascularity is assessed based on the color of the skin and from adequate arterial and venous bleeding from the skin edges.

flap is ultimately divided at the origin of the inferior epigastric artery and vein and prepared for microvascular anastomosis (**Fig. 9.5**). The anterior abdominal wall remains anatomically intact other than the myotomy and anterior sheath incision (**Fig. 9.6**). The microvascular anastomosis is completed using fine sutures or the microvascular coupler (**Fig. 9.7**). Adequate inflow and outflow must be ensured. **Figure 9.8** illustrates a woman following delayed reconstruction of a partial mastectomy deformity using a DIEP flap.

SIEA flap

The SIEA flap is similar to the DIEP flap in that it also utilizes the adipocutaneous component of the lower abdomen. It differs in that there is no myotomy and the anterior rectus sheath is not incised. Its vascularity is derived from the superficial inferior epigastric artery and vein. **Figure 9.9** illustrates a case of a woman with a partial mastectomy deformity that was corrected with a SIEA flap. The preoperative preparation and markings are exactly as with the DIEP flap. The dissection differs from the DIEP flap in that the SIE vessels are identified and dissected towards their origin. The location is usually at the midpoint along the lower abdominal flap between the anterior superior iliac spine and the pubic tubercle. These vessels are not present in all women and sometimes are of poor caliber such that this flap can be performed in approximately 33% of cases. Due to limitations in vascularity, no more than a hemi-flap is recommended. The vessel preparation and microvascular technique are identical to that of the DIEP flap.

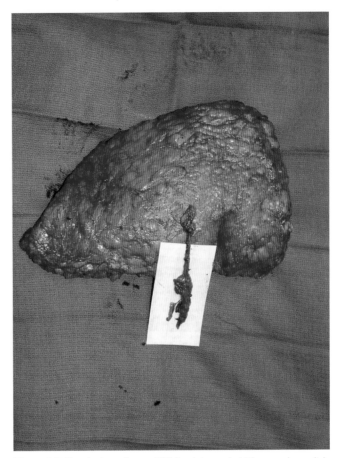

Figure 9.5 The single perforator DIEP flap is harvested. The vascular pedicle ranges from 10 to 13 cm in length and the caliber of the artery and vein ranges from 2 to 3 mm in diameter.

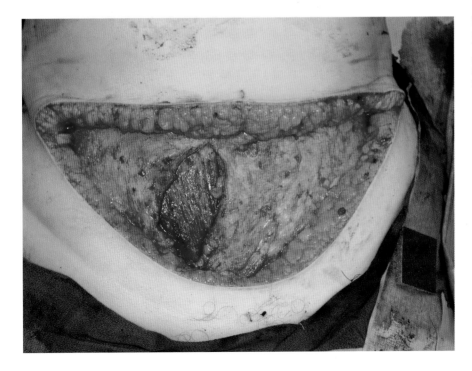

Figure 9.6 The anterior rectus sheath and rectus abdominis muscle are minimally violated. The innervation to the rectus muscle is preserved as is its superior and laterally based blood supply such that the muscle remains innervated and viable.

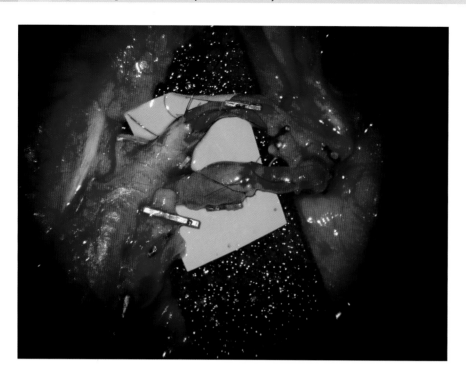

Figure 9.7 Following completion of the microvascular anastomosis, there is excellent inflow and outflow within the perforator flap.

Following completion of the anastomosis, flap inset is completed with a larger skin paddle than the original breast skin deficiency. The flap skin paddle ideally replaces an entire breast aesthetic subunit, rather than leaving a small and poorly concealed patch which is very conspicuous when viewed alongside the native breast skin.[45]

Aesthetic and functional results

When the above measures are incorporated into clinical practice, minimal complication rates can be expected. We have not experienced increased flap failure rates in post-BCT free flap cases. Some patients may develop reactive breast edema which subsides after 6–12 months. Therefore, if further correction is needed, it should be postponed for at least 6 months after the microvascular reconstruction in order to allow these reactive changes to dissipate. A stable aesthetic outcome is usually achieved by 1 year after reconstruction. We would expect better long-term evolution in patients treated with completion subcutaneous mastectomy and free flap replacement, when compared to patients treated with limited partial reconstruction by pedicled flaps, because most of the irradiated tissue has been eliminated.

Surprisingly, many patients express gratitude toward the functional outcome following delayed free flap reconstruction after BCT. They subjectively experience less tightening sensations in their chest wall, and reduced arm edema or heaviness, following microvascular flap transfer to the thorax. We postulate that releasing post-irradiation scar and importing healthy non-irradiated tissue may be responsible for this subjective improvement.

Patient surveillance proceeds on a regular basis, in the same manner as before the surgical correction. Good dialogue between the plastic surgeon, oncologist, and radiologist is essential to following these patients properly. The characteristics of the transferred tissue (fat alone, or muscle and fat combined), and the characteristics of the residual breast tissue (position and amount of retained parenchyma), should be communicated along with any areas of fat necrosis which are identified on postoperative follow-up.

Conclusion

Post-BCT deformity is addressed in a graded manner depending on the degree of deformity, the oncological requirements, and the patient's wishes. Free tissue transfer is an important option for treatment of severe post-BCT deformities. Although the indications are limited, when utilized appropriately it offers superior cosmetic and functional results over other techniques. The potential for microvascular failure remains an important caveat of this demanding technique. The surgeon must remember that the abdominal tissue is the optimal choice for reconstruction of future recurrence or new tumors, and must not be wasted. Careful patient selection, surgical planning, and technical execution are essential to the success of this procedure.

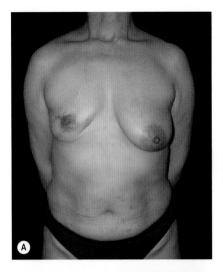

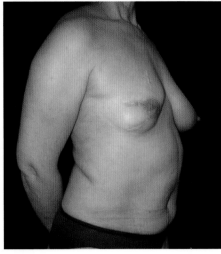

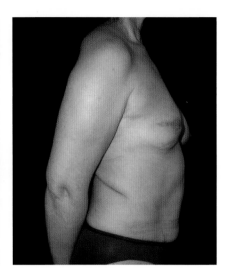

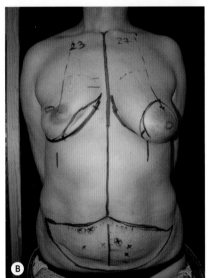

Figure 9.8 A 51-year-old patient who had a conservative breast treatment and multiple previous biopsy procedure in the right breast presented with severe breast deformity. A completed mastectomy was performed with an immediate breast reconstruction using a free DIEP flap. The breast contour deformity in the lower and medial quadrants was restored. (**A**) Preoperative views. (**B**) The plan of surgery: the most damaged breast skin at the lower and medial quadrants was planned for excision. A DIEP flap was designed at the lower abdominal wall and the mapped perforators were also marked preoperatively. The micro-anastomoses were done with the internal mammary vessels. (**C**) The results at 1 year postoperatively.

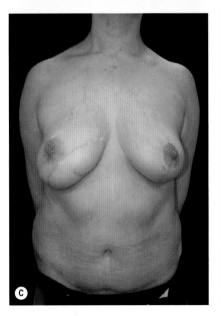

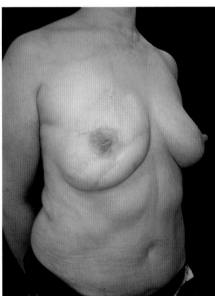

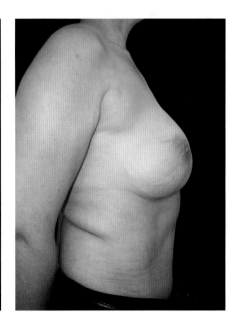

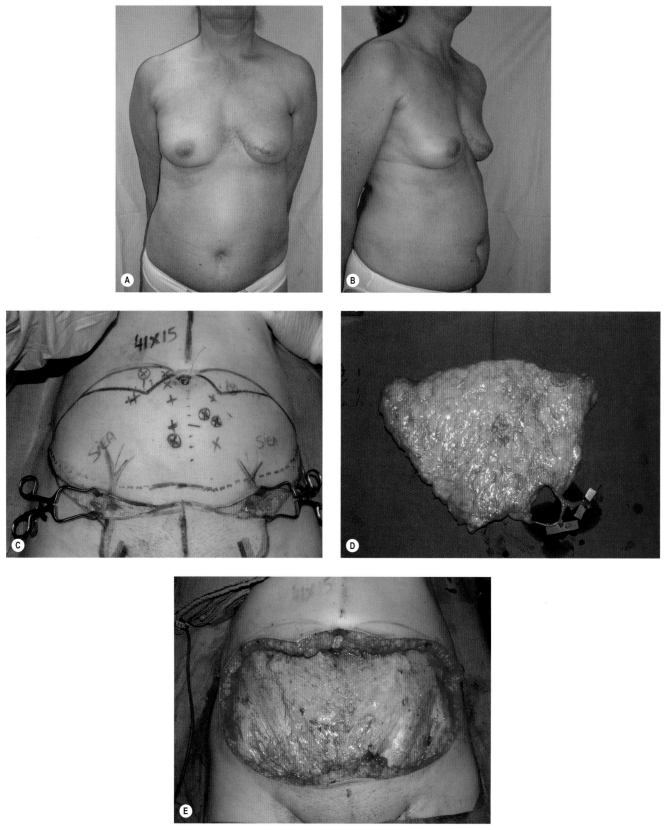

Figure 9.9 A 47-year-old patient presented for a correction of post-BCT deformity on the medial quadrant of left breast and right prophylactic mastectomy with immediate reconstruction. The micro-anastomoses were done to the internal mammary vessels on both sides. (**A**, **B**) Preoperative views. (**C**) Bilateral SIEA flap is planned. SIE vessels are shown with surgical retractors. (**D**) One SIEA flap harvesting. (**E**) The donor site after harvesting bilateral SIEA free flaps.

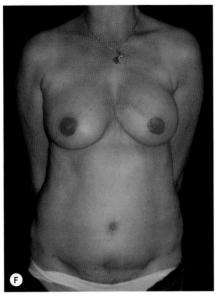 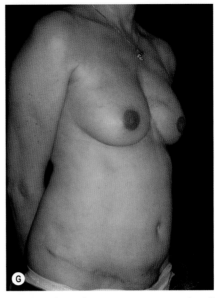

Figure 9.9, cont'd (**F**, **G**) The results at 2 years show good breast symmetry. (M. Hamdi et al. Partial mastectomy reconstruction. Clin Plast Surg 2007; 34(1):51–62).

References

1. Parviz M, Cassel JB, Kaplan BJ, et al. Breast conservation therapy rates are no different in medically indigent versus insured patients with early stage breast cancer. J Surg Oncol 2003; 84:57–62.

2. Veronesi U, Cascinelli N, Mariani L, et al. Twenty-year follow-up of a randomized study comparing breast-conserving surgery with radical mastectomy for early breast cancer. N Engl J Med 2002; 347:1227–1232.

3. Fisher B, Anderson S, Bryant J, et al. Twenty-year follow-up of a randomized trial comparing total mastectomy, lumpectomy, and lumpectomy plus irradiation for the treatment of invasive breast cancer. N Engl J Med 2002; 347:1233–1241.

4. Veronesi U, Banfi A, Del Vecchio M, et al. Comparison of Halsted mastectomy with quadrantectomy, axillary dissection, and radiotherapy in early breast cancer: long-term results. Eur J Cancer Clin Oncol 1986; 22:1085–1089.

5. Arriagada R, Le MG, Rochard F, et al. Conservative treatment versus mastectomy in early breast cancer: patterns of failure with 15 years of follow-up data. Insitut Gustave-Roussy Breast Cancer Group. J Clin Oncol 1996; 14:1558–1564.

6. Fisher B, Redmond C, Poisson R, et al. Eight-year results of a randomized clinical trial comparing total mastectomy and lumpectomy with or without irradiation in the treatment of breast cancer. N Engl J Med 1989; 320:822–828.

7. Poggi MM, Danforth DN, Sciuto LC, et al. Eighteen-year results in the treatment of early breast carcinoma with mastectomy versus breast conservation therapy: the National Cancer Institute Randomized Trial. Cancer 2003; 98:697–702.

8. van Dongen JA, Bartelink H, Fentiman IS, et al. Factors influencing local relapse and survival and results of salvage treatment after breast-conserving therapy in operable breast cancer: EORTC trial 10801, breast conservation compared with mastectomy in TNM stage I and II breast cancer. Eur J Cancer 1992; 28A:801–805.

9. van Dongen JA, Voogd AC, Fentiman IS, et al. Long-term results of a randomized trial comparing breast-conserving therapy with mastectomy: European Organization for Research and Treatment of Cancer 10801 trial. J Natl Cancer Inst 2000; 92:1143–1150.

10. Blichert-Toft M, Rose C, Anderson JA, et al. Danish randomized trial comparing breast conservation therapy with mastectomy: six years of life-table analysis. J Natl Cancer Inst Monogr 1992; 11:19–25.

11. Morrow M, Harris JR. Practice guideline for the breast conservation therapy in the management of invasive breast carcinoma. J Am Coll Surg 2007; 205:362–376.

12. Amichetti M, Busana L, Caffo O. Long-term cosmetic outcome and toxicity in patients treated with quadrantectomy and radiation therapy for early-stage breast cancer. Oncology 1995; 52:177–181.

13. Rose MA, Olivotto I, Cady B, et al. Conservative surgery and radiation therapy for early breast cancer. Long-term cosmetic results. Arch Surg 1989; 124:153–157.

14. Taylor ME, Perez CA, Halverson KJ, et al. Factors influencing cosmetic results after conservation therapy for breast cancer. Int J Radiat Oncol Biol Phys 1995; 31:753–764.

15. Matory WE, Wertheimer M, Fitzgerald TJ, et al. Aesthetic results following partial mastectomy and radiation therapy. Plast Reconstr Surg 1990; 85:739–746.

16. Clough KB, Kroll SS, Audretsch W. An approach to the repair of partial mastectomy defects. Plast Reconstr Surg 1999; 104:409–420.

17. Olivotto IA, Rose MA, Osteen RT, et al. Late cosmetic outcome after conservative surgery and radiotherapy: analysis of causes of cosmetic failure. Int J Radiat Oncol Biol Phys 1989; 17:747–753.

18. Slavin SA, Love SM, Sadowsky NL. Reconstruction of the radiated partial mastectomy defect with autogenous tissues. Plast Reconstr Surg 1992; 90:854–867.

19. Shestak KC. Reconstruction of the radiated partial mastectomy defect with autogenous tissues: discussion. Plast Reconstr Surg 1992; 90:868–869.

20. Kroll SS, Doores S. Nipple centralization for the correction of breast deformity from segmental mastectomy. Ann Plast Surg 1990; 24:271–274.

21. Bold RJ, Kroll SS, Baldwin BJ, et al. Local rotational flaps for breast conservation therapy as an alternative to mastectomy. Ann Surg Oncol 1997; 4:540–544.

22. Clough KB, Cuminet J, Fitoussi A, et al. Cosmetic sequelae after conservative treatment for breast cancer:

classification and results of surgical correction. Ann Plast Surg 1998; 41:471–481.

23. Hamdi M, Wolfli J, Van Landuyt K. Partial mastectomy reconstruction. Clin Plast Surg 2007; 34:51–62.

24. Kroll SS, Schusterman MA, Reece GP, et al. Breast reconstruction with myocutaneous flaps in previously irradiated patients. Plast Reconstr Surg 1994; 93:460–469.

25. Kronowitz SJ, Feledy JA, Hunt KK, et al. Determining the optimal approach to breast reconstruction after partial mastectomy. Plast Reconstr Surg 2006; 117:1–11.

26. Berrino P, Campora E, Santi P. Postquadrantectomy breast deformities: classification and techniques of surgical correction. Plast Reconstr Surg 1987; 79:567–571.

27. Berrino P, Campora E, Leone S, et al. Correction of type II breast deformities following conservative cancer surgery. Plast Reconstr Surg 1992; 90:846–853.

28. Kroll SS, Singletary E. Repair of partial mastectomy defects. Clin Plast Surg 1998; 25:303–310.

29. Chang DW, Kroll SS, Dackiw A, et al. Reconstructive management of contralateral breast cancer in patients who previously underwent unilateral breast reconstruction. Plast Reconstr Surg 2001; 108:352–358.

30. Hamdi M, Van Landuyt K, Monstrey S, et al. Pedicled perforator flaps in breast reconstruction: a new concept. Br J Plast Surg 2004; 57:531–539.

31. Levine JL, Soueid NE, Allen RJ. Algorithm for autologous breast reconstruction for partial mastectomy defects. Plast Reconstr Surg 2005; 116:762–767.

32. Grisotti A, Veronesi U. Reconstruction of the radiated partial mastectomy defect with autogenous tissues, discussion. Plast Reconstr Surg 1992; 90:866–867.

33. Blondeel PN, Beyens G, Verhaeghe R, et al. Doppler flowmetry in the planning of perforator flaps. Br J Plast Surg 1998; 51:202–209.

34. Hamdi M, Van Landuyt K, Van Hedent E, et al. Advances in autogenous breast reconstruction: the role of preoperative perforator mapping. Ann Plast Surg 2007; 58:18–26.

35. Gill PS, Hunt JP, Guerra AB, et al. A 10-year retrospective review of 758 DIEP flaps for breast reconstruction. Plast Reconstr Surg 2004; 113:1153–1160.

36. Granzow JW, Levine JL, Chiu ES, et al. Breast reconstruction with the deep inferior epigastric perforator flap: history and an update on current technique. J Plast Reconstr Aesthet Surg 2006; 59:571–579.

37. Blondeel PN. One hundred free DIEP flap breast reconstructions: a personal experience. Br J Plast Surg 1999; 52:104–111.

38. Hamdi M, Weiler-Mithoff E, Webster M. Deep inferior epigastric perforator flap in breast reconstruction: experience with the first 50 flaps. Plast Reconstr Surg 1999; 103:86–95.

39. Rizzuto RP, Allen RJ. Reconstruction of a partial mastectomy defect with the superficial inferior epigastric artery (SIEA) flap. J Reconstr Microsurg 2004; 20:441–445.

40. Chevray PM. Breast reconstruction with superficial inferior epigastric artery flaps: a prospective comparison with TRAM and DIEP flaps. Plast Reconstr Surg 2004; 114:1077–1083.

41. Hamdi M, Blondeel PN. The superficial inferior epigastric artery flap in breast reconstruction. In: Spear SL, ed. Surgery of the breast, 2nd edn. Philadelphia: Lippincott Williams & Wilkins; 2005:873–881.

42. Yousif NJ, Matloub HS, Kolachalam R, et al. The transverse gracilis musculocutaneous flap. Ann Plast Surg 1992; 29:482.

43. Wechselberger G, Schoeller T. The transverse myocutaneous gracilis free flap: a valuable tissue source in autologous breast reconstruction. Plast Reconstr Surg 2004; 114:69–73.

44. Arnez ZM, Pogorelec D, Planinsek F, et al. Breast reconstruction by the free transverse gracilis (TUG) flap. Br J Plast Surg 2004; 57:20–26.

45. Spear SL, Davison SP. Aesthetic subunits of the breast. Plast Reconstr Surg 2003; 112:440–447.

CHAPTER 10

Repair of the Partial Mastectomy Defect with Staged-Immediate Free Tissue Transfer

Aldona J Spiegel • Liron Eldor

Introduction

Over the last two decades breast-conserving treatment (BCT), consisting of breast-conserving surgery (BCS), radiation therapy (RT), and axillary node sampling, is emerging as the treatment of choice for many women diagnosed with early-stage breast cancer. The aptitude to remove only the necessary amount of breast tissue, leaving as much native breast tissue and skin as possible and judicially leaving the nipple–areola complex (NAC) intact, has revolutionized modern-day treatment of breast cancer. BCT offers women diagnosed with breast cancer the opportunity to maintain the overall breast shape as well as cosmetic, functional, and psychosocial advantages.[1]

Modern prospective studies with follow-up times of up to 20 years have compared mastectomy with BCS and RT for the treatment of early-stage breast cancer (stage I and stage II) and have consistently shown no significant differences in overall or disease-free survival when comparing the two treatments. Furthermore, in recent years a definite reduction in local recurrence rates, with numbers comparing favorably with mastectomy, is achieved using BCT due to more accurate mammographic and pathologic evaluation and, more importantly, the widespread use of systemic therapy. Randomized trials comparing BCT and mastectomy demonstrated similar local recurrence rates, 5.9% versus 6.2%, respectively, and in the more recent trials in which all patients were treated with adjuvant chemotherapy, the 10-year local recurrence rates were lower than 5%.[2]

The growing number of BCT procedures being performed challenges the creativity of the oncoplastic surgeon occasionally confronted with complex three-dimensional partial defects. Reconstruction of partial breast defects resulting from BCT can be broadly categorized into volume displacement techniques versus volume replacement techniques. As a general rule, the ratio of breast mass excision relative to the initial breast volume will assist in choosing between volume displacement and replacement.

Frequently larger breasts (cup C and larger bra size) with smaller excisions are amenable to a variety of described techniques that either reduce and/or rearrange the remaining breast tissue and skin envelope. Often in these situations, manipulation of the contralateral unaffected breast is also required to achieve symmetry. A more challenging task, however, is the partial reconstruction of smaller breasts (cup A and B bra size), which will often require the replacement of volume.

Implementing our gained knowledge with free flap breast reconstruction of total mastectomies utilizing the deep inferior epigastric perforator (DIEP) flap and superficial inferior epigastric artery (SIEA) flap, our group has been performing staged-immediate partial breast reconstruction with mini-SIEA and mini-DIEP flaps. Guided by the rationale of minimizing donor site morbidity while still giving the best reconstructive result we can offer, we believe the abdominal tissue is the most appropriate volume replacement source for our partial free flap reconstructions. We refrain from adding unnecessary scars on the breast and avoid the unsightly back scars, both associated with other techniques.

Although we view the abdominal tissue as the donor site of choice, in cases in which this tissue is unavailable other options exist for free flap reconstructions such as the superior or inferior gluteal artery perforator flaps (SGAP and IGAP), the transverse upper gracilis flap (TUG), and the anterolateral thigh flap (ALT), all of which have mainly been described for total mastectomy reconstruction.

Losken et al published their experience with immediate endoscopic latissimus dorsi flap reconstruction of partial mastectomies at the time of tumor excision based upon initial gross or frozen section analysis. They conclude that although staging the excision and reconstruction raises the cost of initial care, its cautious use might be warranted by the capability to increase patient selection for BCT and improve aesthetic results while preserving oncologic safety.[3] At our institute we postpone the reconstruction until final pathology reports confirm wide negative margins. Reconstruction is staged 7–14 days after initial tumor excision (staged-immediate reconstruction).

The most important aspect when comparing immediate versus delayed reconstruction is the timing of RT. Previous experience with immediate reconstructions of total mastectomies with free flaps and RT has notoriously produced unsatisfactory cosmetic results because of the adverse effects of RT on flaps. In total mastectomy reconstruction, this has led surgeons to defer the reconstruction to a delayed stage.

Contrary to total mastectomies, we have found the effect of RT on mini-flaps to be minute. In fact, even though we recommend harvesting mini-flaps 20% larger as a preemptive measure against flap contracture due to RT effects, we consistently find the flaps to tolerate RT very well and suffer minor contracture, if any (as can be seen in the representative case in **Figs 10.1–10.7**). We attribute the hardiness of mini-flaps to two main factors: first, mini-flaps are essentially smaller flaps that mainly comprise the zone I vascular territory. This produces a higher relation of what we refer to as vascular perfusion territory to flap tissue ratio, meaning hardier perfusion per tissue weight.

Second, the RT protocols for total mastectomies versus partial mastectomies are different; the amount of total

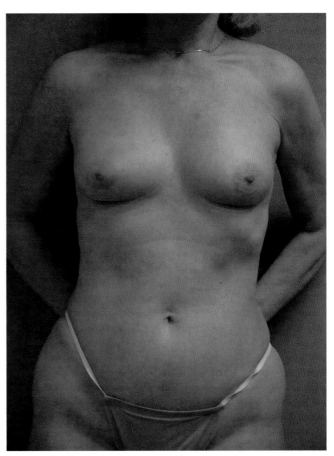

Figure 10.1 Prior to right lumpectomy. 59-year-old female with a strong desire for breast conservation presents with T2 right breast malignancy.

radiation energy is less in BCT, and usually does not include a boost. Thus, logically, the damage to the flap itself and surrounding skin is expected to be much smaller in partial mastectomies.

In our institute the RT protocols are as follows:
- BCT: 4500 cGy in 25 fractions with a daily dose of 180 cGy; patients occasionally receive boost.
- Total mastectomy: 5040 cGy in 28 fractions with a daily dose of 180 cGy; patients receive boosts of 200 cGy for a total of 1000 cGy in five fractions.

The advantages of staged-immediate reconstruction with mini-flaps are:
- Operating in a non-irradiated field with hardier tissue perfusion and no post-irradiation fibrosis and scarring.
- Immediate positioning of the flap provides a scaffold and minimizes skin contracture and breast tissue collapse that is often seen in delayed reconstruction, thus simplifying the accurate recreation of the excisional defect and more precise flap tailoring.
- A smaller skin island is required, which in most cases can be reduced or even completely removed at a later stage.

- Diminishes psychological distress from the partial mastectomy, shortening the time period the patient has to live with the excisional deformation.
- Improved cosmetic result in breast contour and skin sensation.
- Improved sensation and positioning of the nipple areola-complex.

Indications, contraindications, and patient selection (Table 10.1)

One of the most important factors in patient selection is the patient's desire to preserve native breast tissue, principally the NAC.[4] Patients showing high motivation

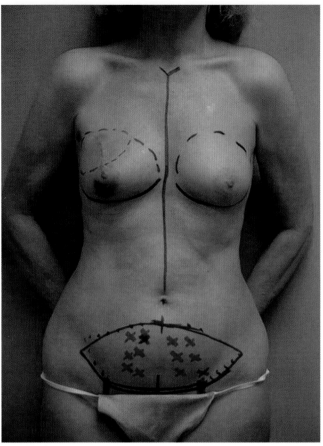

Figure 10.2 Preoperative markings. Note the outline of the seroma cavity on the right breast and the low design of the flap on the abdomen. Several inferior perforators of the DIEA are included in the flap design.

Table 10.1 Indications and contraindications for patient selection

Indications	Contraindications
Stage I, II breast cancer	Advanced-state breast cancer
Small–medium-sized breast	BRCA 1 and BRCA 2 positive
Remaining breast is negative for	patient
suspicious lesions per MRI	Suspicious MRI findings
Patient motivated to undergo BCS	Unfavorable cancer oncotype
and RT	Active smoker
Patient willing to continue with	Concomitant high-risk
periodic radiological follow-up	surgical morbidities
Slightly elevated BMI with excess	Positive microscopic tumor
abdominal tissue	margins
Negative microscopic tumor margins	

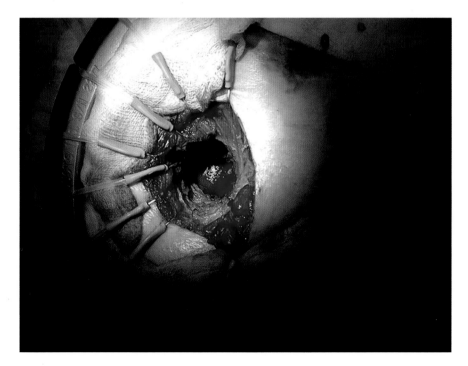

Figure 10.3 Intraoperative. Dissection of internal mammary perforator recipient vessels.

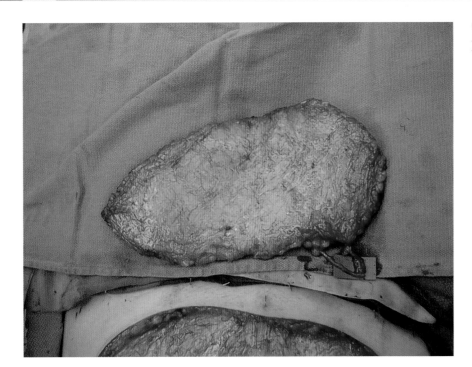

Figure 10.4 Intraoperative. Right mini-SIEA flap after harvest prior to shaping. Note the SIEA and vena comitans (laterally) and the SIEV (medially).

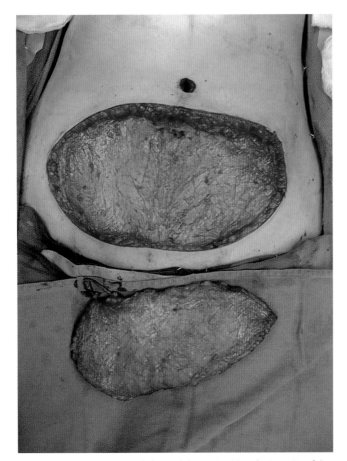

Figure 10.5 Intraoperative. Abdominal donor site. Note the integrity of the anterior rectus sheet. The umbilicus has been released and closure of donor site is about to commence.

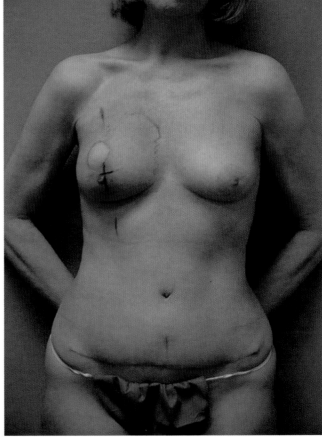

Figure 10.6 Postoperative. Right mini-SIEA flap during radiation therapy treatment.

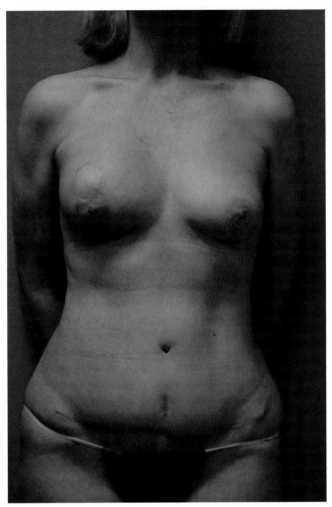

Figure 10.7 Postoperative. One-year follow-up after BCT with staged-immediate partial breast reconstruction using a mini-SIEA flap. Patient deferred revisional surgery for symmetry and skin paddle reduction. Note low-lying, bikini-line, well-healed abdominal donor scar and small well-healed vertical abdominal scar.

towards conservation therapy will be more willing to undergo a more extensive free tissue transfer of a muscle-preserving flap, accept the unavoidable donor site scar, comply with the pre- and postoperative instructions, and most importantly, conform to the needed periodic physical and mammographic evaluations.

One aspect in which partial breast reconstruction is different from total mastectomy reconstruction is the amount of tissue needed for reconstruction. The amount of excess abdominal tissue required is usually much smaller in partial reconstructions; hence the ideal patient need not have large amounts of excess abdominal tissue. Owing to the design of the mini-SIEA and mini-DIEP flaps, the ideal body habitus should be normal to slightly elevated body mass index (BMI), and mild to moderate lower abdominal wall laxity, as is often seen after pregnancies.

In our experience, patients perceive the sacrifice of lower abdominal tissue as an added cosmetic bonus to

their cancer treatment and are willing to accept the well-hidden lower abdominal scar. Frequently, the lower abdominal scar is merely an extension of an already existing Pfannenstiel scar. Several studies have demonstrated high patient satisfaction rates with abdominal contour subsequent to lower abdominal perforator flap harvest for breast reconstruction.[5,6]

Exclusion criteria include patients with advanced-stage cancer, BRCA 1 and BRCA 2 positive patients, large-breasted women (cup D or larger bra size), very thin patients with no abdominal tissue excess or redundancy, suspicious magnetic resonance imaging (MRI) findings, positive microscopic tumor margins, and concomitant high-risk surgical morbidities.

The following is a list of relative contraindications we use for all our free tissue transfers to the breast: active smoking history, age greater than 60 years, BMI greater than or equal to 35 kg m^{-2}, prior abdominal surgery with extensive scarring, prior abdominal liposuction, and coagulation disorder.

Preoperative history and considerations

In our institute only early-stage breast cancer patients are candidates for staged-immediate partial breast reconstruction. Prior to surgery patients should undergo a preoperative physical evaluation and mammography (preferably MRI) to rule out any other suspicious lesions on the same breast as well as the contralateral side.

The preoperative physical examination and mammographic studies are not only important for staging but are also helpful in assessing the ratio of expected tissue excision relative to the size of the breast, and the resulting breast deformity. In a study conducted by Cochrane, cosmesis and satisfaction after BCS correlated with the percentage of breast volume excised.[7] This ratio is fundamental not only in choosing to proceed with BCT versus mastectomy, but also in choosing the appropriate reconstructive strategy. As previously mentioned, a smaller excision in a large breast will most probably prompt for local rearrangement or reduction techniques, while bigger excisions on small to medium-sized breasts negate the addition of tissue into the breast.

Since there is always a possibility for incomplete initial tumor excision with microscopically involved margins or sentinel node involvement, we preferentially defer the reconstructive surgery. As this is a staged-immediate reconstruction, the reconstructive surgery is carried out only after the final pathology is reviewed. For all intents and purposes, we attempt to stage the partial breast reconstruction with free flaps within 2 weeks after cancer excision and axillary node sampling. This time frame allows for thorough review of the pathological specimens, tumor staging, and final decisions on treatment protocol.

Only patients that have negative microscopic tumor margins of at least 1.0 cm are offered abdominal free tissue transfer.[8,9] This latter criterion highlights one of the major advantages of free tissue transfer for BCT: the abundance of tissue available for reconstruction, offering the oncologic surgeon the opportunity to perform wide-margin excisions without hesitation regarding resultant skin and volume deformity. In this regard, another recommendation is to have the oncologic surgeon clip mark the excisional cavity in case re-excision is indicated.

The excised specimen's size, weight, and location should also be recorded during the excisional stage and taken into consideration during the reconstructive phase. We prefer to use a flap that is approximately 20% larger than the excised specimen to compensate for possible flap contracture and changes due to the irradiation treatment. Also, accurate location of the excised specimen is vital for choosing the appropriate recipient vessels since the flap is routinely anastomosed to a perforator vessel at the nearest vicinity to the excisional defect (this point will be discussed under surgical technique).

Operative approach

Surgical anatomy

The mini-SIEA flap is perfused by the superficial epigastric artery, which originates approximately 1–3 cm below the inguinal ligament from the common femoral artery. The SIEA originates as either an independent trunk in roughly 40% of the cases, or shares a common trunk with the circumflex iliac artery in almost 50% of the cases, with various other variants of origin from the deep femoral artery and pudendal artery in the remaining dissections. The length of the main pedicle (artery and two vena comitans) can vary from 8 to 15 cm, with an additional superficial inferior epigastric vein (SIEV) lying medially to the main pedicle.[10]

In our series of over 300 clinical dissections, the SIEA was absent or inconsequential in 42% of total dissections. In the remaining 58%, only half of the SIEA had an external diameter greater than or equal to 1.5 mm at the level of the lower abdominal incision. This latter criterion is the norm when we apply our previously described algorithm for use in the SIEA flap in total breast reconstructions where the recipient vessel is the internal mammary artery.[11] Since the recipient vessels in our partial reconstructions are perforator vessels (as will be discussed later under choosing recipient vessels), we often use SIEA with an external diameter of 1.3 mm or more. The better size match between the recipient perforator vessel and the donor vessel is one of the reasons we preferably use the mini-SIEA flap in staged-immediate partial breast reconstructions.

The mini-DIEP flap is perfused by the deep inferior epigastric artery (DIEA), which originates directly from the terminal part of the external iliac artery or, rarely, as a common trunk with the obturator artery. The DIEA has an average pedicle length of 10.3 cm (range 9–13 cm).[12] In the majority of cases, the DIEA provides cutaneous perforators from medial and lateral branches, with the latter being the dominant system. The number of cutaneous perforators with a diameter of 0.8 mm or more ranges from one to three on each hemi-abdomen, with the majority concentrated within a radius of 8 cm from the umbilicus. A key factor in the surgical anatomy of the mini-DIEP flaps is the inclusion of lower perforator vessels in the lower abdominal flap design. These inferior perforators are usually smaller in diameter compared to their periumbilical counterparts.

Preoperative marking and preparation

On the day of surgery, the patient is marked using a handheld Doppler. Initially, marking is done in the supine position. We begin by marking the superficial abdominal vascular system, locating the superficial inferior epigastric artery with its vena comitans and the superficial inferior epigastric vein located medially to the artery. Next, the deep vascular network is marked by tracing the location of both the medial and lateral perforator rows.

Since the mini-flap donor site is located on the lower part of the abdomen, an important aspect of perforator location when using mini-DIEP flaps is the marking of inferior perforators (contrary to the traditional superior periumbilical perforators marked in standard DIEP flaps).

Next, we mark the flap; the lower incision is placed just above the pubic hair line and is carried out laterally with a gentle sloping curve to the anterior superior iliac spine (ASIS). When planning a mini-SIEA flap, it is crucial to keep a low incision line as the diameter of the SIEA increases proximally towards its origin. The proposed upper incision line is then chosen, taking into account both the existing abdominal tissue laxity and the anticipated amount of tissue needed for reconstruction. In slimmer-bodied patients, the upper incision line might be located below the umbilicus, thus necessitating a small, low vertical scar produced due to the relocation of the umbilicus. Patients should be educated and consented regarding this scar.

We continue marking with the patient standing up; first outlining the lumpectomy defect, then marking the inframammary folds, midline, sternal notch, and conclude by measuring the abdominal incision lines for symmetry.

In the operating room, the patient is positioned supine with arms tacked to the sides, prepped from the neck to the upper thighs, and draped, leaving the shoulders, chest, abdomen and pubis exposed. In cases where a lateral defect is reconstructed, the ipsilateral arm should also be prepped and extended on an arm-board to facilitate dissection of the recipient serratus perforator vessels.

Re-creation of the excisional defect and exposure of the recipient vessels

It is imperative that the initial step in the operation be the recreation of the lumpectomy defect and preparation of the recipient vessels for anastomoses. When attempting to recreate the excisional defect, a key point is careful dissection and awareness of any perforator vessels in the vicinity. Particularly when using the mini-SIEA flap, perforators encountered in the dissection are carefully clamped and spared as they might be of suitable size match to the flap vessels. Any existing scars or non-viable tissues are removed, as is any apparent serous cavity lining. Once the excisional cavity is re-created, a template is drawn on sterile glove paper to be duplicated later at the donor site.

One of the biggest advantages in using free flaps for the staged-immediate reconstruction is the opportunity to choose a recipient vessel in the vicinity of the defect, thus allowing flexibility in the orientation of both flap pedicle and the added tissue.

Depending on the location of the defect, we will preferentially choose a branch of the following arteries: serratus, thoracodorsal, thoracoacromial, or internal mammary. We attempt to spare the internal mammary artery in the event that future reconstructive attempts will warrant its use; but if necessary we will access it at the level of the second, third, or fourth intercostal space.

Flap dissection

As previously noted, the lower abdominal incision is carried out just above the pubic hair line and extended laterally in a curvilinear fashion towards the ASIS. Keeping in mind that the flap design has to allow for dissection of either the superficial or deep inferior epigastric vascular networks, one should not 'burn bridges' during initial flap dissection until a decision has been made. The skin incision is carefully made just to the subcutaneous level, taking care not to incise the SIEA or SIEV. With the mini-SIEA flap being our first choice, the SIEA is first explored bilaterally. If an appropriate vessel exists, with an external diameter of at least 1.3 mm at the height of the incision line, and there is a visible, palpable, and audible (Doppler) pulse, we will then continue with the dissection of the mini-SIEA flap. Both ipsilateral and contralateral flaps can be used, depending on donor vessel adequacy and preferred flap inset orientation. The SIEA is traced proximally into the femoral foramen while its vena comitans are dissected proximal to their point of convergence. The SIEV is dissected and carefully clipped for potential venous anastomosis; nonetheless, we will preferentially use the vena comitans owing to their proximity to the artery, which typically produces a superior length match.

As mentioned previously, the superior incision is made taking into consideration both the amount of tissue needed for reconstruction and the available abdominal tissue laxity. Once the inferior and superior incisions are made, harvest of the SIEA flap is carried out quite rapidly in a suprafascial plane from lateral to medial. The template of the excisional defect is then traced onto the flap, choosing both the preferred pedicle and donor tissue positioning. The vasculature is then clipped, and the donor flap transferred to the breast.

In cases in which the SIEA has been deemed inappropriate, we will proceed with reconstruction using the mini-DIEP flap. As previously mentioned, it is critical to include the lower perforators in the flap design. We prefer to include two perforators in the mini-DIEP flap design owing to the smaller size of these inferior perforators.

The mini-DIEP flap is harvested in a suprafascial plane from medial to lateral until the lateral row of perforators is reached. A decision is then made regarding the quality of these vessels. Either the anterior rectus sheath is longitudinally incised around the lateral perforators and the lateral branch dissected, or the dissection proceeds to explore the medial row perforators. Dissection of the vascular pedicle proximally commences until a suitable length and vessel diameter are obtained to match the recipient vessels.

Flap inset and closure

The flap is oriented in the appropriate position in relation to the recipient vessels and vessels are anastomosed. We routinely use an anastomotic coupler for the vein and also the artery in cases in which smaller, more elastic perforator arteries are coupled. In larger, less compliant arteries, we use a running 9/0 nylon micro suture. As in all our free flap cases, an internal venous Doppler is placed around the recipient vein proximal to the anastomosis. The internal venous Doppler signal quality and intensity are noted prior to and following final flap inset, to ensure compression or kinking of the vessels has not occurred.

Once flap perfusion is achieved, we commence with the delicate task of flap tailoring and inset into the defect. Zone III, VI and any other questionably viable tissues are discarded, leaving a flap that is at least 20% larger than the defect size. The skin paddle is marked appropriately (again, about 20% larger) and any excess is de-epithelialized accordingly.

The flap skin paddle is temporarily anchored to the surrounding breast skin with staples and the patient flexed to a seated position. The breasts are then assessed for symmetry and any contour irregularities on the reconstructed side are marked. The bed is then returned to a horizontal position to facilitate closure of the abdomen. Any final adjustments in flap positioning and contour are made, and the flap is finally anchored to the surrounding breast tissue as needed, using absorbable sutures. Prior to skin closure, drains are placed in the breast, avoiding the vicinity of the fresh anastomosis. Skin is finally closed with interrupted subdermal absorbable sutures and a continuous intradermal suture.

Abdominal closure is performed with the bed flexed to relieve tension on the abdominal flaps. In cases in which a mini-DIEP was harvested, the rectus fascia is closed with non-absorbable sutures. Any existing diastasis recti or hernia is repaired at this stage, and two drains are introduced and secured laterally. The umbilicus is delivered through a neo-umbilical opening; occasionally a small vertical scar exists due to transposition of the umbilicus. In selected patients with a high waistline and lax abdominal tissue, transposition of the umbilicus is not necessary, thus the umbilicus is left attached or floated as described for mini-abdominoplasty. Next, the cut sides of Scarpa's fascia are re-approximated, followed by the subdermal and dermal layers.

Optimizing outcome

- High-power magnification (5.5× loupe magnification) is always essential for atraumatic perforator dissection of both donor and recipient vessels. Mishandling of these vessels may lead to intraluminal microtrauma, predisposing the vessels to thrombosis.
- Vessel coupling devices are used liberally as they help reduce flap ischemia time and total operative time. Since the majority of free flap partial breast reconstructions are done using both donor and recipient small-diameter perforator vessels, coupling is used for both veins and arteries.
- Tailoring of the recipient vessel closest to the area of reconstruction is paramount in achieving a tension-free contoured flap inset. For medial and central defects the internal mammary perforator vessels are our first choice. The thoracodorsal and serratus perforators are more suited for lateral defects.
- When choosing the flap dimensions one should expect flap shrinkage due to RT. It is beneficial to design a flap that is approximately 20% larger than the re-created excisional defect. If indicated, flap dimensions and skin paddle can be reduced as a second revisionary stage.
- After RT we recommend that any revisions to the flap be done mostly as an excisional procedure using minimal judicious liposuction, since in our experience irradiated flaps are less tolerable of liposuction.
- Internal Doppler monitoring of the venous flow is highly beneficial and sensitive in detecting early patency concerns. Moreover, since only a small skin pedicle is used it is often impossible to locate an external Doppler signal.
- Regarding the lumpectomy defect, first, it is important to recreate the defect to its full extent;

second, preparing a template of the defect cavity is helpful in designing the flap.
- Final flap positioning and shaping should be done in the sitting position with the patient's arms tucked at the sides.
- Although we believe the mini-SIEA is the flap of choice in partial staged-immediate reconstructions, one should use caution in selecting vascular pedicles with appropriate external diameters. As noted previously, since the vascular anastomosis is usually between matching size perforator vessels, we are more lenient toward using SIEA with an external diameter of less than 1.5 mm at the lower abdominal incision site. However, we do not encourage the use of SIEA smaller than 1.3 mm or vessels that do not exhibit a visible palpable pulse with an audible Doppler signal.
- We highly recommend the inclusion of more than one of the inferior perforators in the mini-DIEP flaps.
- Whenever venous drainage is questionable and flap congestion is suspected, we recommend augmenting venous drainage by adding a second venous anastomosis connecting the SIEV to a matching vein in the vicinity.

Complications and side effects

Total or partial flap loss

Flap perfusion is monitored vigorously with the use of the internal Doppler, capillary refill testing, and an external Doppler when possible. Any suspicion of vascular compromise is promptly managed with a very low threshold for surgical re-exploration of the anastomosis. In instances where excess edema is noticed in the flap and/or surrounding breast, intravenous dexamethasone is administered and skin sutures may be removed. In our institute, a dedicated nursing staff was educated in the special requirements of post-reconstructive monitoring, handling, and patient care. This dedicated team allows expert management of these more demanding cases.

Deep vein thrombosis (DVT)

DVT prophylaxis is routine using low-molecular-weight heparin (Lovenox®) monitored with thromboelastogram viscoelastic testing. Intermittent compression devices are applied from surgery to discharge, and the patient is mobilized at an early stage.

Fat necrosis

Fat necrosis is uncommon in our experience with mini flaps. Careful excision of all poorly perfused tissue and gentle flap inset should minimize areas of fat necrosis. Any suspicious lumps or bumps should be visualized, preferentially with an MRI, and biopsied accordingly.

In the adverse event of total flap loss or cancer recurrence necessitating completion mastectomy, other free flaps are available for reconstruction. Flaps from the gluteal and thigh region become a valid option and can usually be anastomosed to either the internal mammary or thoracodorsal vessels (both remaining unaffected due to use of recipient perforators for previous anastomosis). Depending on the amount of tissue needed, one may also choose local or regional flaps such as the thoracodorsal artery perforator (TAP) flap, lateral thoracic flap, or latissimus dorsi flap with or without an implant.

Postoperative care

For the immediate postoperative care, the patient is transferred to the intensive care unit for the first 24 hours, allowing close nurse monitoring of the patient and the flap on an hourly basis. In our institute, a dedicated nursing staff was educated in the special requirements of post-reconstructive monitoring, handling, and patient care. This dedicated team allows expert management of these more demanding cases. On postoperative day one, the patient is transferred to the floor, allowing gradual ambulation. Patients are discharged home on postoperative day three or four, depending on individual progress.

The patient is instructed to minimize ipsilateral arm elevation higher than 60 degrees and to avoid excess arm exertion starting immediately after surgery for a period of 2 weeks. We recommend all patients sleep on a recliner for 3 weeks to prevent accidental lying on the reconstructed side and compression of the vascular pedicle.

Anticoagulation prophylaxis is initiated after surgery using low-molecular-weight heparin and monitored with thromboelastogram viscoelastic testing according to a treatment protocol we have formulated. Ketorolac is added to the anticoagulation prophylaxis or is used to replace the low-molecular-weight heparin as needed. The patient is discharged from the hospital with a baby aspirin prescription.

Secondary revisions of the flap are usually postponed until after the completion of RT. It is advisable to wait at least 6 months post completion of RT prior to revising the flap. As mentioned previously, the irradiated flaps are much less tolerant of liposuction than the non-irradiated; hence, we recommend mainly excisional revisions with minimal judicious liposuction. At this stage we also address any breast asymmetry by ipsilateral revisions and/or contralateral mastopexy, reduction, or augmentation.

In cases in which there is evident excess of the skin paddle, we offer to partially reduce or even totally excise the skin paddle, leaving a smaller paddle or only a linear scar. To date, none of the patients have sought revision of the skin paddle.

Life-long oncologic surveillance is mandatory in patients who undergo BCT. As mentioned under patient selection, the patient must be highly motivated to preserve the remaining breast and NAC and to commit to this demanding life-long monitoring. We recommend the use of MRI as the standard for subsequent breast surveillance.

Conclusion

With the increasing popularity of BCS, more and more women diagnosed with early-stage breast cancer are being offered immediate partial breast reconstruction. In experienced hands, good to excellent aesthetic results can be achieved in the majority of cases. In our institute, over 90% of total breast reconstructions are done with free transfer of abdominal tissue, as SIEA or DIEP flaps. With the gained expertise, we have begun using mini-SIEA and mini-DIEP flaps for staged-immediate breast reconstruction as part of BCT.

When questioned regarding their aesthetic results, most patients convey high satisfaction with the surgical outcome regarding both the reconstructed breast and the abdominal donor site.

We believe the mini-SIEA and mini-DIEP flaps are a welcome addition to the reconstructive surgeon's arsenal. Future creative approaches will broaden the application of these and other free flaps in partial breast reconstruction.

References

1. Clough KB, Thomas SS, Fitoussi AD, et al. Reconstruction after conservative treatment for breast cancer: cosmetic sequelae classification revisited. Plast Reconstr Surg 2004; 114(7):1743–1753.
2. American College of Radiology. Practice guideline for the breast conservation therapy in the management of invasive breast carcinoma. J Am Coll Surg 2007; 205(2):362–376.
3. Losken A, Schaefer TG, Carlson GW, et al. Immediate endoscopic latissimus dorsi flap: risk or benefit in reconstructing partial mastectomy defects. Ann Plast Surg 2004; 53(1):1–5.
4. Wellisch DK, Schain WS, Noone RB, et al. The psychological contribution of nipple addition in breast reconstruction. Plast Reconstr Surg 1987; 80:699–704.
5. Nahabedian MY, Tsangaris T, Momen B. Breast reconstruction with the DIEP flap or the muscle-sparing (MS-2) free TRAM flap: is there a difference? Plast Reconstr Surg 2005; 115(2):436–444.
6. Wolfram D, Schoeller T, Hussl H, et al. The superficial inferior epigastric artery (SIEA) flap: indications for breast reconstruction. Ann Plast Surg 2006; 57(6):593–596.
7. Cochrane RA, Valasiadou P, Wilson AM, et al. Cosmesis and satisfaction

after breast-conserving surgery correlates with the percentage of breast volume excised. Br J Surg 2003; 90(12):1505–1509.

8. Freedman G, Fowble B, Hanlon A, et al. Patients with early stage invasive cancer with close or positive margins treated with conservative surgery and radiation have an increased risk of breast recurrence that is delayed by adjuvant systemic therapy. Int J Radiat Oncol Biol Phys 1999; 44:1005–1015.

9. Smitt MC, Nowels KW, Zdeblick MJ, et al. The importance of the lumpectomy surgical margin status in long-term results of breast-conserving. Cancer 1995; 76(2):259–267.

10. Ninkovic M. Superficial inferior epigastric artery perforator flap. In: Blondeel P, Morris S, Hallock G, eds. Perforator flaps: anatomy, technique and clinical applications, Vol I. St Louis, MO: Quality Medical Publishers; 2006:405–419.

11. Spiegel AJ, Khan FN. An intraoperative algorithm for use of the SIEA flap for breast reconstruction. Plast Reconstr Surg 2007; 120(6):1450–1459.

12. Heitmann C, Felmerer G, Durmus C, et al. Anatomical features of perforator blood vessels in the deep inferior epigastric perforator flap. Br J Plast Surg 2000; 53(3):205–208.

Nipple-Sparing Mastectomy and Reconstruction: Indications, Techniques, and Outcomes

Scott L Spear • Catherine M Hannan

Introduction

Nipple-sparing mastectomy (NSM), or subcutaneous mastectomy, combines a skin-sparing mastectomy with preservation of the nipple–areola complex (NAC), with the possibility of intraoperative pathological assessment of adjacent tissue. Immediate reconstruction after NSM may allow for a better cosmetic result for patients undergoing total mastectomy. However, because of the impossibility of removing all glandular and ductal tissue from beneath the NAC, the oncologic safety of this procedure continues to be questioned.

Subcutaneous mastectomy for primary breast cancer or risk reduction has been described for several decades. In 1962, Freeman[1] pioneered this surgical procedure, but it was eventually discredited because of unclear selection criteria, poor cosmetic results, high rate of complications, and lingering questions about its oncologic safety or efficacy. For the majority of the 20th century, removal of the NAC complex has been a standard part of a mastectomy, despite the fact that the nipple is a relatively uncommon site for breast cancer to develop.[2] The most often observed neoplasia of the nipple is Paget's disease of the breast (intraepidermal tumor cells of the nipple), which remains an uncommon presentation of breast malignancy, accounting for 1–3% of all breast tumors.[3] Nipple involvement may also occur in association with ductal carcinoma in situ (DCIS) or invasive breast cancer in the breast parenchyma. Fortunately, however, carcinoma of the nipple is extremely rare.[2] Meanwhile, with the advent of screening protocols allowing for earlier breast cancer detection and therefore smaller tumors and lesser-stage cancers, it has become increasingly tempting to preserve more and more of the native breast skin, leading to the classic 'skin-sparing mastectomy'.

With ever-increasing expectations of improved cosmetic results from breast reconstruction, it would only seem natural that nipple-sparing mastectomy would become the next consideration. It has the potential to remove virtually all glandular tissue similar to other mastectomies, yet preserve the NAC, as is done with breast-conserving procedures. It needs to be emphasized, however, that regardless of mastectomy technique, including modified radical mastectomy, it is impossible to completely remove 100% of breast tissue.

If the use of nipple-sparing mastectomy is questionable because of the possibility of an increased risk of local recurrence in the nipple area, this procedure may be more acceptable in the prophylactic setting. In that setting, nipple-sparing mastectomy has been shown to dramatically reduce the incidence of breast cancer in high-risk patients.[4]

Indications

1. Prophylactic/risk reduction mastectomy.
2. Nipple-sparing mastectomy in the treatment of breast cancer.

Risk reduction mastectomy

The concept of NSM was first popularized in the 1960s and 1970s as subcutaneous mastectomy.[5] That procedure for risk reduction quickly fell out of favor for a number of good reasons. Most significantly, there were no scientifically based selection criteria and therefore no possibility of ever demonstrating efficacy. Beyond that, the reconstructive techniques of the day were relatively crude, the results were inconsistent, the best outcomes were not impressive, the complication rate was high, and a significant amount of breast tissue was intentionally left behind.

All this changed with the seminal report by Hartmann et al,[6,7] published in the *New England Journal of Medicine* on January 14, 1999. Over the preceding 20 years or longer, the Mayo Clinic in Rochester, Minnesota, had been a center of sorts for prophylactic mastectomy where the techniques were largely of the historic subcutaneous mastectomy type, but where the medical records were excellent and data could be extracted and reassessed using computer models and other more modern techniques. The data from that series of 639 women demonstrated that prophylactic mastectomy did indeed have a protective benefit, reducing the risk of breast cancer in both high-risk and moderate-risk groups by 81–94%. Ninety percent of the mastectomies in that series were nipple-sparing of the subcutaneous variety. Breast cancer developed in seven women after prophylactic mastectomy. Six cancers were confined to the chest wall at diagnosis and were specifically not in the area of the NAC. One patient in the high-risk group presented with bone marrow metastases from adenocarcinoma with no evidence of breast disease. There was no statistically significant difference in the cancer-preventing benefit whether the nipple was removed or retained.[8]

In the context of risk reduction, other series report similar experience. McDonnell et al,[9] also from the Mayo Clinic, reported in 2001 in the *Journal of Clinical Oncology* on a series of 745 women with a first breast cancer and a strong family history of breast cancer who underwent unilateral prophylactic mastectomy between 1960 and 1993, resulting in a projected 94–96% risk reduction. All told, there were eight breast cancers versus 156 predicted. Forty-one percent of the mastectomies spared the nipple, while 59% did not. The eight cancers that developed were evenly split, four and four, between the nipple-sparing and nipple removal groups. None of the eight cancers that did occur developed near the nipple.

In 2004, Crowe[10] reported on 17 nipple-sparing prophylactic mastectomies performed from 2001 to 2003. They recommend a lateral incision for improved nipple–areola survivability. There were no occult cancers seen on frozen or permanent examination beneath the nipple and no cancers have developed since.

In 2006, Sacchini[11] published in the *Journal of the American College of Surgeons* a larger multi-center experience including the Memorial Sloan-Kettering Cancer Center in New York and major cancer centers in Sao Paulo (Brazil), Milan, and Padua (Italy). Altogether there were 55 patients who underwent nipple-sparing prophylactic mastectomies. There were no recurrent or new cancers in the nipple with mean follow-up of 24 months. Two cancers did develop after prophylactic mastectomy: one in the axillary tail 24 months postoperatively and one in the upper outer quadrant at 62 months. The majority of their nipple-sparing procedures were performed via a periareolar incision, which included coring out the nipple. Twenty-two out of 192 nipples suffered some degree of necrosis, nine of which resulted in loss of more than one-third of the NAC.

TR Rebbeck et al[12] published a combined multi-center experience from the Prose study group of 483 BRCA 1 and 2 positive women, 105 of whom underwent bilateral prophylactic mastectomy, including 29 nipple-sparing. Two of those 105 developed breast cancer, in contrast to 184 cancers among 378 patients in the control group, yielding a 90% or more risk reduction. The two cancers that developed included one in the axilla and one in the breast. There was no statistically significant difference in the occurrence of cancer between the nipple-sparing and non-nipple-sparing groups.

Nipple-sparing mastectomy in the treatment of breast cancer

If surgeons have been reluctant to embrace NSM in the context of risk reduction, then they have been even more reluctant to do so in the face of established breast cancer. Nevertheless, the gradual acceptance of skin-sparing mastectomy has encouraged some to look more critically at the concept of NSM as a treatment for breast cancer in order to better define inclusion criteria, exclusion criteria, preoperative strategies, operative strategies, surgical technique, and overall value.

There were many inconsistent reports from the 1970s and 1980s regarding the likelihood of nipple involvement with cancer in the face of known ipsilateral breast cancer. Reports of nipple involvement with cancer varied widely from 0 to 58%. Much of that data comes from reports in the 1970s and 1980s based upon examination of the mastectomy specimens from an era of later diagnosis and more advanced disease. Further, the methodology for tissue examination of those studies and the criteria for describing 'involvement' were not uniform.

With the increased interest in skin-sparing mastectomy and even NSM, more relevant studies have recently been done. Christine Laronga et al[13] from the MD Anderson Cancer Center in Houston reported in 1999 on

326 patients whose breasts were examined after skin-sparing mastectomy. They described how earlier studies correlated a greater risk of occult NAC involvement with the primary tumor being close to the NAC, larger than 2 cm, poorly differentiated, and associated with positive axillary lymph nodes. They found 16 (5.6%) instances of occult tumor involvement. They believe four of these would have been identified on frozen section if it had been done. The only statistically significant predictors of nipple involvement were location (subareolar or multicentric) and axillary nodal status. The authors speculate that their finding of a relatively low incidence of occult NAC involvement might reflect their selective preoperative criteria for NSM in the first place. They conclude that it would be appropriate to offer NAC preservation in axillary node negative patients with tumors located on the periphery of the breast. They estimate that in that group the probability of missing occult tumor in the NAC would be less than 2%.

Bernd Gerber and colleagues[14] from Rostock, Germany, reported in the *Annals of Surgery* in 2003 their experience with skin-sparing mastectomy, including conservation of the NAC. At 59 months, there were six (5.4%) recurrences in 112 nipple-sparing mastectomies: two on the chest wall, two in the upper breast, one in the fold, and one non-invasive in the nipple. There were 11 (8.2%) recurrences among 134 women who had the nipple removed. They found NAC tumor involvement depended predominantly on the distance of the tumor to the NAC. They believe that their data justify preservation of the NAC in patients with preoperatively evaluated tumors at least 2 cm from the nipple, no extensive intraductal component (extensive defined as greater than 25%), and intraoperatively demonstrated clear margins.

Crowe[5] at the Cleveland Clinic attempted NSM in 54 women from September 2001 until June 2003. Frozen section findings of disease in the nipple resulted in aborting the procedure in six patients. Of the 48 women who underwent NSM, three had partial nipple loss. Candidates for NSM were excluded if the tumor was 3.5 cm in diameter or greater, if the tumor was central, if the patient had undergone neoadjuvant chemotherapy, and if there was inflammatory breast cancer or Paget's disease. Overall, they recommended lateral incisions whenever possible. Of note even with their exclusion criteria, of 37 patients who underwent NSM for cancer, six (16%) had neoplastic involvement based upon frozen section.

In Sacchini's[6] report of a multi-center, multinational experience with NSM in 68 patients with breast cancer, they excluded women with very large breasts, very ptotic breasts, and tumors within 1 cm of the areola. Fourteen patients of the original 82 were excluded and not included among the remaining 68 because of tumor involvement found on permanent pathological evaluations. They did not employ frozen sections in their series, and thus finding occult nipple involvement with tumor was only possible on permanent pathologic review.

More recently, Laura Esserman and colleagues[15] from San Francisco described their experience with total skin-sparing mastectomy (nipple-sparing mastectomy) in 64 breasts in 43 women. Twenty-nine breasts were prophylactic and 24 were for invasive cancer or DCIS. They recommended high-resolution magnetic resonance imaging (MRI) with fat suppression to exclude tumor within 2 cm of the nipple. Nevertheless, even with MRI screening two occult cancers were found on frozen section. Further, they do not recommend NSM in cases with large, centrally located tumors, skin involvement by tumor, or MRI evidence of tumor within 2 cm of the nipple.

Of similar interest is the recommendation by Govindarajulu and colleagues[16] from Bristol, UK, to screen patients for possible NSM by performing preoperative ultrasound-guided mammotome assessment. Thirty-three women had 36 procedures, and seven of the 36 had a positive biopsy. The histopathology of the mastectomy specimen correlated 100% with the mammotome biopsy.

Discussion: operative approach and optimizing outcomes

It is clear from a review of the literature of the last 15 years that the subject of NSM is complex and evolving. The subject is properly divided into two parts: risk prevention and therapeutic mastectomy. There now seems little doubt that NSM is an oncologically safe approach to prophylactic mastectomy. For this purpose, proper patient selection and technique remain open questions. In the case of prophylactic mastectomy, it is therefore not whether NSM is oncologically safe, but how to do it and for which patients. The larger or more ptotic the breast, the more complex the planning. Strategies for saving the nipple in these more challenging cases could include reducing the skin envelope prior to the mastectomy, grafting the NAC, or performing a mastopexy at the same time as the mastectomy.

NSM at the time of therapeutic mastectomy remains more controversial. There is a developing consensus by those interested in NSM as a possibility with therapeutic mastectomy that it is best suited for women who meet certain criteria. On clinical assessment, they ideally should have tumors 3 cm in diameter or less, 2 cm away from center of the nipple, clinically negative axillae or sentinel node negative, no skin involvement, and no inflammatory breast cancer. If possible, they should have a preoperative MRI of the breast to further exclude nipple involvement. Alternatively, or in addition, they might benefit from preoperative ultrasound-guided mammotome biopsy of the tissue beneath the nipple. In any case, the final decision to spare the nipple must ultimately await frozen and then definitive pathologic section. This is with the caveat of an accepted false negative rate for frozen section, in which case the decision to remove the nipple would be deferred until the more definitive permanent pathology returns.

Assuming that all the oncologic criteria are met in the patient with breast cancer, the issues come back to patient selection and technique. In that regard the answers are the same or similar as with prophylactic mastectomy. In evaluating the oncologic criteria for NSM, it is obvious that it is not the ideal solution for every patient because the risk of occult tumor involvement overall has been reported to be as high as 50%. But that 50% figure is for all breast cancers without selecting out lower-risk patients. From the many recent studies that have looked at this subject more carefully, certain basic preoperative criteria can lower the risk of occult tumor in the nipple substantially. The collective data suggest that, using the criteria of tumor less than 3 cm in diameter, tumor more than 2 cm from the center of the nipple and clinically negative nodes, or perhaps negative sentinel node biopsy, the risk of occult tumor in the nipple should be 5–15%; further, that frozen section of the base of the nipple will identify many if not most of those occult tumors; and finally, that the risk of occult tumor in patients screened as above with frozen section negative findings is low, with a 4% or so false negative rate from frozen section.[17]

The ability to diagnose breast cancer at an earlier stage and to stage it more accurately using simple criteria enhanced with MRI, improved mammography, and possibly even preoperative subareolar mammotome biopsy, should allow surgeons to offer NSM to the properly screened patient with a high level of confidence of not finding occult disease. If occult disease is encountered on frozen or permanent pathology examination then the nipple and perhaps the areola should be removed, at the time of surgery or at a later date in the case of a false negative frozen section and positive nipple at the time of permanent pathology.

Although selection criteria can be used to identify patients at lower risk for occult tumor in the nipple, it should not be inferred that other patients cannot be considered if they desire. It does mean that they are at higher risk for having occult cancer in the nipple, resulting in removal of the nipple at the time of mastectomy or shortly thereafter.

NSM is not meant to be the solution for the patient who is a poor candidate for breast conservation, because many of those same patients would also be poor candidates for NSM. Rather, it is meant to be an option for the patient who wants to retain all the surface landmarks of the breast and forgo radiation therapy.

Selection criteria must also include the anatomy of the breast itself. In most cases, NSM equates with removing little if any skin. For that reason, the larger or more ptotic the breast, the more likely there will be nipple or flap necrosis, or both. A plastic surgeon should screen possible candidates for NSM to make certain that it is technically realistic. In cases where the skin flaps would be too long, then the NAC could be harvested and grafted onto a flap, preferably a latissimus or transverse rectus abdominis myocutaneous (TRAM) flap.[8] Such flap and NAC graft combinations are highly complex efforts, best practiced by very experienced teams.

Regarding technique, recent reports suggest that the best incisions are either lateral, radial, lateral mammary fold (LMF), inframammary fold (IMF) or in any case do not traverse more than one-third of the areola diameter. The IMF incision is not recommended except for very small breasts, because of several concerns including safe access to the upper portion of the breast.[5]

Optimizing outcomes

Patient selection (reconstructive criteria)

- Very large or ptotic breasts may not be candidates (may consider free nipple grafts on latissimus or TRAM).

Patient selection (oncologic criteria)

- Tumors < 3 cm.
- Tumors at least 2 cm from the nipple.
- Absence of significant multifocal or multicentric disease.
- No skin involvement or inflammatory breast cancer.
- Clinically negative axillae or negative sentinel node.
- Negative preoperative MRI or tissue immediately beneath or within the nipple.
- Possible preoperative ultrasound-guided mammotome biopsy of the ducts.

Operative technique

Preferred incisions are lateral, radial, or LMF. IMF is less preferable as it is more difficult to access the upper breast and manage the nipple when disease is present there:

- Intraoperative frozen section of the retro-nipple tissue – if positive, nipple is not retained
- Reconstructive options are diverse.

Figures 11.1–11.6 illustrate clinical outcomes following NSM and immediate reconstruction using either prosthetic devices or autologous tissues.

Complications

The potential complications most relevant to this procedure are those of partial or complete nipple loss, nipple malposition on the breast, as well as delayed involvement of the nipple with cancer. In light of the accepted false negative rate of frozen sections, if the permanent pathology returns with cancer at the base of the nipple, the nipple and/or entire NAC should be removed. In the series reported thus far, the rate of nipple necrosis has not been appreciably higher than that of other known complications of mastectomy and reconstruction, such as seroma, infection, hematoma, or fat necrosis. Careful preoperative planning of mastectomy incisions as well as

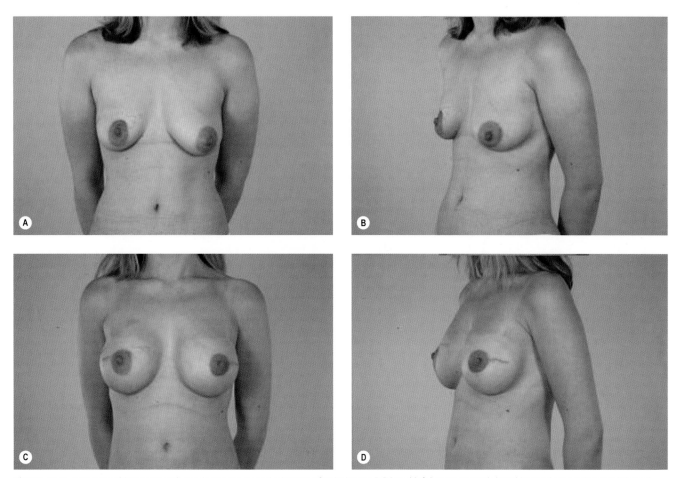

Figure 11.1 A 27-year-old woman with moderate ptosis and a history of right breast DCIS and left breast atypical ductal hyperplasia underwent bilateral NSM with immediate tissue expander reconstruction. Subsequently, expanders were exchanged for shaped silicone gel filled textured implants.

gentle manipulation of the flaps intraoperatively may prevent these potentially serious sequelae.

In a study by Nahabedian et al in 2004 examining the outcomes and complications of NSM and immediate reconstruction, 14 breasts were analyzed in 12 patients, 11 of which were therapeutic for cancer. Reconstruction included both implant and autologous with latissimus, free TRAM or deep inferior epigastric artery perforator. Postoperatively, sensation was present in six of 14 nipples, (42.9%), delayed wound healing occurred in four of 14 breasts (28.6%), one of which involved the nipple itself, symmetry with the contralateral breast was achieved in five of 10 women (50%) after unilateral reconstruction, tumor recurrence was noted in three of 11 breasts (27.3%), and secondary procedures related to the NAC were necessary in five of the 14 breasts (35.7%). Outcomes were graded as excellent in three, good in eight and poor in three breasts.[18] Despite variability in the aesthetic outcomes, patient satisfaction tends to be very high when retaining the nipple.

In a recent study by Spear et al which is currently pending publication, the complications and outcomes of reconstruction after prophylactic mastectomy were compared with those of therapeutic mastectomy. With a mean follow-up of 31 months, there was only one breast site complication in 28 breasts that underwent NSM: a unilateral mastectomy skin flap necrosis. More significantly, when combined with all skin-sparing mastectomies, there were more breast-site complications in reconstructions following mastectomy for cancer when compared with the prophylactic side, although this difference was not statistically significant. Moreover, when the patients were surveyed, the results from reconstruction after prophylactic mastectomy trended towards improved aesthetic outcomes compared with reconstruction after therapeutic mastectomy. Theoretically, these differences can be attributed to the fact that women with breast cancer are more likely to undergo chemotherapy and an increasing number are having post-mastectomy radiation. Furthermore, prophylactic mastectomy can be considered inherently elective in nature. The timing is elective, the choice of reconstruction technique is entirely elective, and the choices for incision and the options for nipple-sparing or areola-sparing are almost always available. The luxury of being an elective procedure provides the widest possible latitude in counseling patients, selecting patients, planning incisions, and choosing the reconstructive techniques. Such latitude could provide the opportunity for somewhat improved results, lower risk, and higher satisfaction.[19]

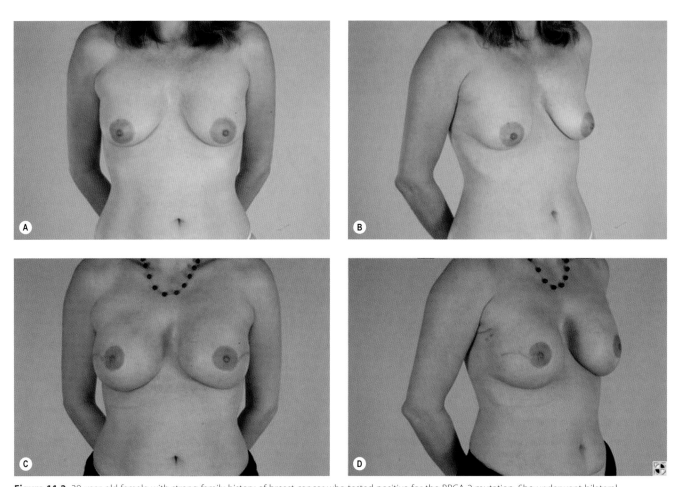

Figure 11.2 39-year-old female with strong family history of breast cancer who tested positive for the BRCA 2 mutation. She underwent bilateral prophylactic NSM with immediate tissue expander reconstruction. Subsequently, expanders were exchanged for silicone gel filled round implants.

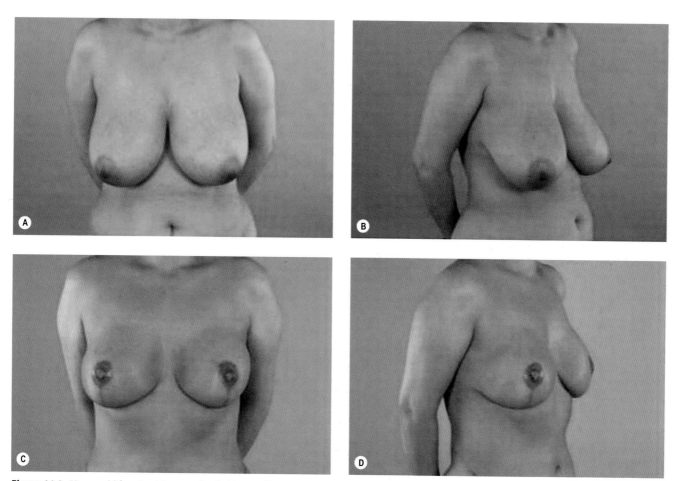

Figure 11.3 53-year-old female with strong family history of breast cancer and severe ptosis who underwent bilateral prophylactic mastectomies with free nipple grafts which were banked on bilateral pedicled TRAM flaps. As a final stage, she underwent bilateral delayed mastopexies.

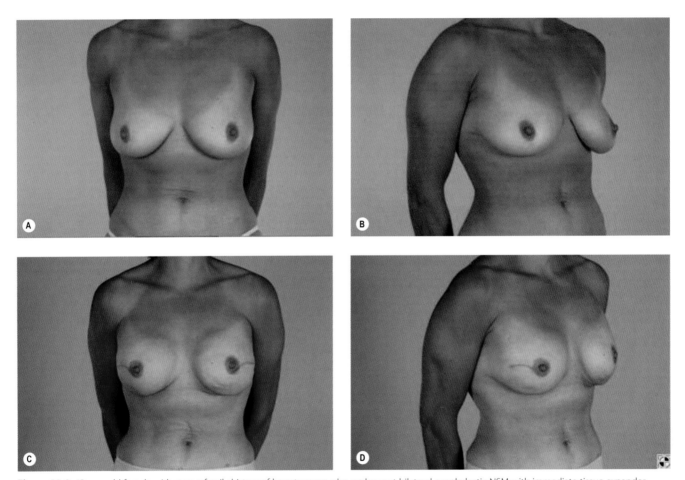

Figure 11.4 42-year-old female with strong family history of breast cancer who underwent bilateral prophylactic NSM with immediate tissue expander reconstruction. The expanders were then exchanged to smooth round silicone gel filled implants.

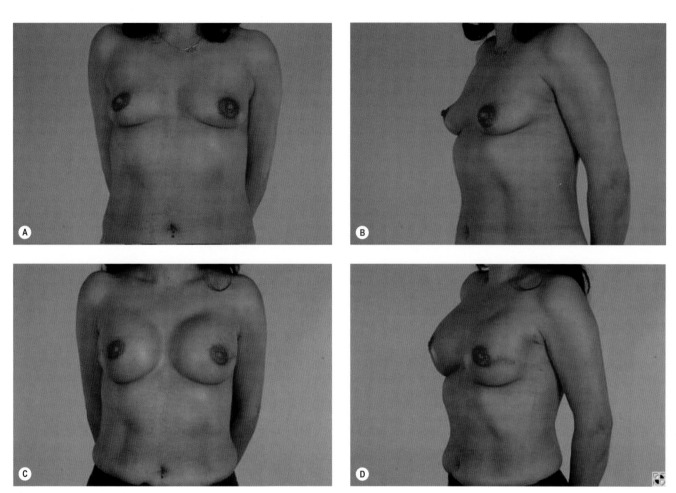

Figure 11.5 44-year-old female with strong family history of breast cancer who tested positive for BRCA 2 mutation. The patient underwent bilateral prophylactic mastectomy with immediate tissue expander reconstruction. These were exchanged to round silicone gel implants.

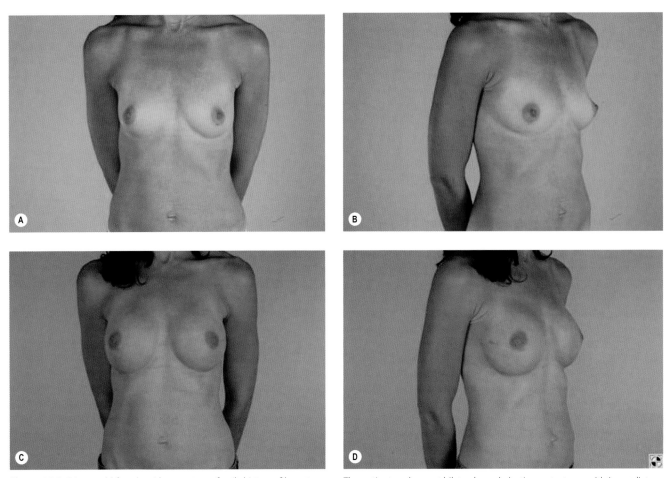

Figure 11.6 36-year-old female with very strong family history of breast cancer. The patient underwent bilateral prophylactic mastectomy with immediate tissue expander reconstruction. These were exchanged to round silicone gel implants.

Conclusions

Based on our patient selection criteria and operative technique, we feel that NSM is a safe and effective technique. Reconstructive techniques include prosthetic devices or autologous tissues. Results have been good to excellent, with high patient satisfaction. This option should be included within the armamentarium of the ablative and reconstructive surgeon.

References

1. Sacchini V. Nipple-sparing mastectomy for breast cancer and risk reduction: oncologic or technical problem? J Am Coll Surg 2006; 203(5):704–714.
2. Chen C, Sun L, Anderson B. Paget disease of the breast: changing patterns of incidence, clinical presentation, and treatment in the US. Cancer 2006;107(7):1448–1458.
3. Caliskan M, Gatti G, , et al. Paget's disease of the breast: the experience of the European Institute of Oncology and review of the literature. Breast Cancer Res Treat 2008; Feb 1.
4. Hartmann LC, Sellers TA, Schaid DJ, et al. Efficacy of bilateral prophylactic mastectomy in BRCA 1 and BRCA 2 gene mutation carriers. J Natl Cancer Inst 2001; 93:1633–1637.

5. Freeman BS. Subcutaneous mastectomy. Plast Reconstr Surg 1962; 30:676–682.
6. Hartmann LC, Schaid DJ, Woods JE, et al. Efficacy of bilateral prophylactic mastectomy in women with a family history of breast cancer. N Engl J Med 1999; 340(2):77–84.
7. Hartmann LC, Sellers TA, Schaid DJ, et al. Efficacy of bilateral prophylactic mastectomy in BRCA 1 and BRCA 2 gene mutation carriers. J Natl Cancer Inst 2001; 93(21):1633–1637.
8. Spear S, Carter ME, Schwarz K. Prophylactic mastectomy: indications, options, and reconstructive alternatives. Plast Reconstr Surg 2005; 115(3):891–909.

9. McDonnell SK, Schaid DJ, Myers JL, et al. Efficacy of contralateral prophylactic mastectomy in women with a personal and family history of breast cancer. J Clin Oncol 2001; 19(19):3938–3943.
10. Crowe JP. Nipple-sparing mastectomy: technique and results of 54 procedures. Arch Surg 2004; 139(2):148–150.
11. Sacchini V. Nipple-sparing mastectomy for breast cancer and risk reduction: oncologic or technical problem? J Am Coll Surg 2006; 203(5):704–714.
12. Rebbeck TR, Friebel T, Lynch HT, et al. Bilateral prophylactic mastectomy reduces breast cancer risk in BRCA 1 or 2 mutation carriers: the Prose Study Group. J Clin Oncol 2004; 22:1055–1062.

13. Laronga C, Kemp B, Johnston D, et al. The incidence of occult nipple–areola complex involvement in breast cancer patients receiving a skin-sparing mastectomy. Ann Surg Oncol 1999; 6(6):609–613.

14. Gerber B, Krause A. Skin-sparing mastectomy with conservation on the nipple-areola complex and autologous reconstruction is an oncologically safe procedure. Ann Surg 2003; 238(1):120–127.

15. Wijayanayagam A, Kumar AS, Foster RD, et al. Optimizing the total skin-sparing mastectomy. Arch Surg 2008; 143(1):38–45

16. Govindarajulu S, Narreddy S, Shere MH, et al. Preoperative mammotome biopsy of ducts beneath the nipple areola complex. Eur J Surg Oncol 2006; 32(4):410–412.

17. Vlajcic Z, Zic R, Stanec S, et al. Nipple–areola complex preservation predictive factors of neoplastic nipple–areola complex invasion.

Ann Plast Surg 2005; 55:240–244.

18. Nahabdian M, Tsangaris TN. Breast reconstruction following subcutaneous mastectomy for cancer: a critical appraisal of the nipple–areola complex. Plast Reconstr Surg 2006; 117(4):1083–1090.

19. Spear S, Schwarz K, Venturi M, et al. Prophylactic mastectomy and reconstruction: clinical outcomes and patient satisfaction. Plast Reconstr Surg 2008; 122(1):1–9.

Oncoplastic Breast Surgery and the Effects of Radiation Therapy

Navin K Singh • Anu M Singh

Background

Breast cancer is one of the most common cancers and the second leading cause of cancer mortality in US women. Breast malignancy accounts for nearly one in three cancers diagnosed in women in the United States. Hence much attention and resources have been directed at this disease – from attempts at prevention, to screening, treatment, and cure. Approaches range from the infinitesimal to the global, analyzing molecular markers of gene expression such as HER-2/neu, genetic-based testing and screening such as BRCA 1 and 2, familial analyses, hormonal assays, population studies, and vaccine trials.

While the incidence of breast cancer continues to increase, fortunately mortality is starting to decline because of earlier detection prior to distant spread, attributable to the unequivocal success of mammographic screening efforts, as well as advances in management. With approximately 182 000 cases expected in 2008, the public health impact estimates are between $5 and $8.1 billion dollars annually spent on managing breast cancer. This expansive clinical volume has created a body of evidence that has been gathered, reviewed, published, and disseminated, leading to a decline in mortality from breast cancer over the last few decades.

Owing to research efforts directed at breast cancer, breast management has undergone significant evolutions in management – from the Halsted radical mastectomy to the modified radical mastectomy to breast conservation therapy combined with radiation. Paralleling these paradigmatic changes in oncologic management have been shifts and changes in the reconstructive algorithms to reconstruct breast cancer defects, whether they be mastectomy or partial defects.

To maximally benefit the patient with breast cancer seeking treatment, the complex interplay of radiation and plastic surgery must be thoroughly understood to offer the most appropriate treatments in the most appropriate sequence with the best anticipation of the likely outcomes. This requires an understanding of the physics, mechanisms of action of radiobiology, and pathophysiology associated with radiation and with wound healing.

The goals for oncoplastic breast surgery and radiation are (1) tumor eradication, (2) prolonging survival, and (3) maximizing quality of life via cosmetically acceptable breast preservation, or breast reconstruction to a close facsimile of the original. Data from the Early Breast Cancer Trialists' Collaborative Group (EBCTCG) indicate that not only is there improvement in local control, but also an absolute survival benefit of approximately 5% in women who receive radiation.

Oncoplastic breast management exists at the nexus of four disciplines – surgical oncology, plastic surgery, radiation oncology, and medical oncology – and the timing, efficacy, and role of each of these modalities must be considered concomitantly. Often a tumor board or multi-disciplinary breast center is a good forum to brainstorm and create a management plan which resonates with the expertise that is brought to bear from each specialty and with the patient's goals, expectations, lifestyle, and particular tumor grade, histopathology, stage, genetics, and oncotype in mind.

Role of radiation

Radiation therapy has two principal roles in the management of breast carcinoma. It can be combined with lumpectomy as part of breast-conserving therapy (lumpectomy + XRT) or be utilized as adjuvant treatment for post-mastectomy treatment (PMRT). The specific removal of a breast tumor with an adequate margin is interchangeably called lumpectomy, quadrantectomy, or tumorectomy. The discussion in this chapter is limited to these two roles, although radiation might be used for palliation to mitigate symptomatology from an incurable lesion such as ulceration, bleeding, or pain either in the breast or at a metastatic site.

Basic science and biology

Radiation therapy is the use of ionizing energy to control malignancy. The energy (interpretable as high-speed particles or electro-magnetic waves) is targeted to the tumor and a surrounding zone of normal tissue to kill cancer cells preferentially.

The unit of measurement in radiation is the gray (Gy), the absorbed dose of 1 joule of radiation energy by 1 kilogram of matter, and may be used to denote any type of radiation. It does not describe the biological effect of that 1 joule in that 1 kilogram. The sievert (Sv) describes the biologically equivalent dose by a multiplier Q for the quality of radiation. For gamma and X-radiation, both of which are types of photons, $Q = 1$ and a sievert is equivalent to a gray:

$$\text{One gray } [1\,\text{Gy} = 1\,(\text{J/kg}) = 1\,\text{m}^2\,\text{s}^{-2}] \text{ is equivalent to 100 rads}$$

Radiation is administered for adjuvant purposes (that is, when all known detectable disease has been resected) in breast cancer, and occasionally in palliation as well. It is not used with curative intent as the sole modality. Gamma rays and electrons are used commonly, but X-rays are never utilized in therapeutic radiation oncology.

Radiation fields include a surrounding zone of normal tissue to control for tumor motion such as respiro-phasic motion or shift of skin marker alignment, variation in motion, and daily set-up. The ionizing injury from radiation serves to cause irreparable damage to the DNA of rapidly dividing cells – typically malignant cells since they lack an intact repair mechanism. Some collateral damage is suffered by other rapidly dividing cells such as

epithelial structures. During the simulation phase of treatment planning, relatively fixed points of skin are tattooed to help align the radiation portal. A significant proportion of women may want these excised after XRT is completed, but they should be encouraged to retain these so that overlapping fields of XRT can be avoided should future contralateral radiotherapy be needed.

A typical treatment course is 5 days a week for 5–6 weeks for a total radiation dose of 5000 cGy (50 Gy) to the entire breast by tangential beams to eradicate microscopic disease, with a boost to the tumor bed of approximately 1000–2000 cGy (10–20 Gy). There is fairly solid consensus about the utility of the local boost, and the European Organization for Research and Treatment of Cancer (EORTC) has reported on improved local control with a boost since most recurrences are seen at the primary site. This fractionation, called postoperative fractionated radiotherapy, remains the standard method for conservative treatment of breast carcinomas.

Typical results in breast radiation are mild signs of skin changes and mild volume asymmetry related to atrophy and lumpectomy resection, as seen in **Figure 12.1**.

The collateral damage to non-cancer dividing cells causes both the acute sequelae and the long-term sequelae of radiation. Short-term sequelae include skin edema, which typically disappears in 12–24 months. Skin adnexal structures such as sebaceous glands and hair follicles may be irreversibly lost, causing dry skin and fissuring. The incidence of radiation dermatitis is as high as 90%, although the majority of instances are relatively mild and well tolerated. Treatment is supportive via the use of antibiotics, emollients, and analgesics. Dry desquamation arises from XRT damaging the basal stem cells in the deep layer of the epidermis, which create the cornified layer of the epidermis. It is shedding of the cornified layer. If the

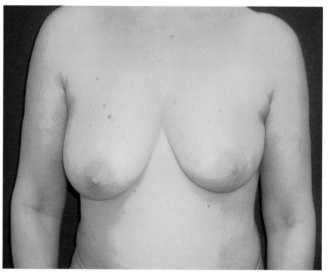

Figure 12.1 Patient underwent left BCT with radiation therapy and had a cosmetically salutary result with only subtle differences from the contralateral breast. She developed a recurrence, years later.

basal layer is further destroyed and the dermis is exposed, then moist desquamation develops.

Morbidity is exacerbated in obese patients, diabetics, smokers, and those with previous radiation.

Long-term sequelae are progressive atrophy, telangiectasias, hyperpigmentation, impeded wound healing because of loss of precursor cells in a radiated field, fibrosis, and loss of volume (**Fig. 12.2**). Lymphedema may occur from either axillary dissection or from fibrosis of lymphatic channels post radiation (**Fig. 12.3**). It may involve the chest wall or arm. Higher at risk are the obese and those with full axillary clearance. The incidence of lymphedema approaches approximately 9–14%. Treatment is compression garments and avoiding procedures

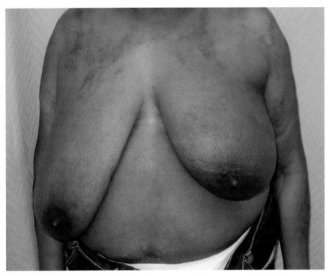

Figure 12.2 This woman was likely not an ideal candidate for BCT and would have benefited from an oncoplastic breast reduction with lumpectomy initially. She presented after lumpectomy and radiation therapy on her left breast, with complaints of asymmetry.

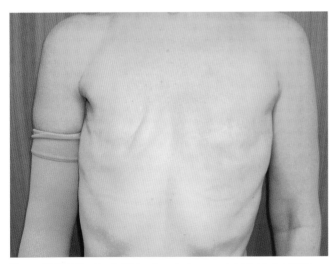

Figure 12.3 Patient is s/p bilateral mastectomy and right sided radiation. Right-sided lymphedema related to radiation and lymph node dissection is managed conservatively with compression garments.

in the affected arm such as blood pressure measurements and phlebotomy. Conservative measures such as compression stockings, and manual lymphatic drainage, suffice. Rarely, lymphatic reconstruction or bypasses can be done using microvascular techniques.

Skin hyperpigmentation arises from superficial migration of melanocytes and may be permanent after a few years. Fatigue is common. Rib weakening or fractures may occur, especially with tissue expanders being constrained by indurated skin. Fractures can be diagnosed by plain film or bone scan. A pathologic fracture related to bony metastasis must be ruled out. Treatment is conservative, allowing the bone to heal with rest and supportive measures.

Pain and limitation in range of motion at the shoulder may be related both to the surgical resection, axillary dissection, and radiation. Physical therapy is routinely prescribed and most patients regain the full range of their routine motions.

Induced malignancy may develop post radiation, and may occur as frequently as 7–8%. Studies indicate a 1% absolute increase in second non-breast malignancies associated with XRT, such as lymphangiosarcoma, lung cancer, and sarcomas.

Radiation pneumonitis may develop in 1–7% of patients and is manifested as a dry cough and/or low-grade pyrexia. Pericarditis and coronary damage remain largely theoretical concerns. There are concerns that radiotherapeutic treatment of the left breast (and left-sided breast cancer is slightly more common than right-sided breast cancer) can cause coronary fibrosis and sclerosis. This was seen with older technologies, and current planning techniques minimize the coronary risk of radiation. The risk bears mentioning, especially since many chemotherapeutic regimens used to manage breast cancer deliver cardiotoxic medications as well (e.g., adriamycin and herceptin). Further, breast reconstruction with a free flap may harvest the internal mammary vessels as donor vessels, and render them inaccessible for future coronary revascularization – a theoretical limitation since much coronary artery disease is treated via angioplasty, stents, or vein grafts. While breast cancer is the most common cancer in women, the leading cause of mortality in US women is still coronary artery disease.

Breast-conserving treatment

Indications

Overall, 65% of breast cancers are classified as early stage (1 and 2) and three-quarters are eligible for BCT, or about half of all breast cancers. Of those that are eligible for BCT, about 20% choose to have a mastectomy.

In 1985, NSABP-B06 (The National Surgical Adjuvant Breast and Bowel Project) demonstrated that BCT provides equivalent 5-year survival rates when compared with modified radical mastectomy for the treatment of early breast cancer. BCT rates range from 10% to 50% of eligible patients, and depend on a plethora of factors such as referral patterns, presence of a multidisciplinary team, education level of patients, and prevailing cultural norms. Patient satisfaction rates range from 75% to 95% but many women note significant asymmetries. Up to 30% may benefit from corrective surgery. In addition to randomized control trials comparing lumpectomy + XRT with mastectomy, there are good randomized trials comparing lumpectomy alone with lumpectomy and radiation. Lumpectomy has a local recurrence rate of 30–40% at 5 years, which drops to 10% when combined with radiation. A recent meta-analysis of 10 randomized trials showed an absolute reduction in recurrence rates of approximately 17% with radiation. The cultural zeitgeist now is overwhelmingly breast preservation.

- *Early-stage tumor.* Randomized controlled trials have demonstrated the safety for Stage 1 and 2 tumors. Even certain Stage 3 tumors, depending largely on tumor size, are candidates for BCT.

- *Small tumor.* There is theoretically no upper limit on size, so long as negative margins can be obtained through a non-deforming excision. However, larger tumor volumes may be considered unsuitable because of concerns for margins. Further imaging is indicated to rule out other foci of disease, and additional image-guided biopsies may be needed to address the matter conclusively before proceeding with BCT.

- *Unifocal disease.* Previously, an extensive intraductal component (EIC) was felt to be a poor prognosticator for the success of BCT; however, so long as margin control is obtained during lumpectomy, unifocal disease, even with an EIC, is an indication for BCT. EIC was first described by the Joint Center for Radiation Therapy as DCIS with an invasive component or DCIS comprising 25% of an invasive tumor with DCIS in surrounding parenchyma. It no longer precludes BCT.

- *Patient preference.* The patient must be motivated to preserve the breast. Most patients who are candidates for BCT do opt for it; however, a fifth of the eligible patients opt for a mastectomy.

- *Previous cosmetic breast augmentation.* Prior augmentation mammaplasty is not a contraindication, and the implants do not have to be removed. This applies equally to whether the implants are submuscular or subglandular.

Contraindications

Certain conditions make BCT untenable because of unacceptable consequences associated with radiation. While every rule has its exception, there is broad consensus in the following contraindications. Some of these are relative contraindications in view of the caveats mentioned.

- *Inability to obtain uninvolved margins.* Certain tumors may be extensive enough or close enough to the chest wall that adequate clearance with negative margins is not feasible with a lumpectomy. When all detectable disease cannot be eradicated, then BCT is not offered.

- *Inadequate cosmesis.* The goal of BCT is breast conservation, and so if the likely outcome of a lumpectomy is going to be distortion and poor cosmesis, patient dissatisfaction is likely (**Fig. 12.4**). Particularly when a small breast with a proportionately large resection is anticipated, mastectomy might be a more palatable alternative. Other situations where disappointing appearance is likely are subareolar position of the tumor or where the excision will create a poor scar orientation. A recent study shows that approximately 25% of women who have undergone BCT + XRT will be sufficiently displeased with the aesthetic outcome as to warrant a plastic surgery referral. Axillary dissection did not impact the cosmetic outcome.

- *Prior radiation.* If portions of the chest or breast have been previously radiated for breast cancer or received mantle radiation (e.g., for Hodgkin's lymphoma), then the woman is ineligible for BCT + XRT. If total body dose is likely to be exceeded, then the patient is also ineligible for BCT. Should the total tolerable dose of the breast, skin, and chest wall be exceeded, skin breakdown, ulceration, and irreversible radiation injury may result. Additional, focal radiation might be considered in certain specific scenarios nevertheless.

- *Locally advanced tumors or inflammatory breast cancer.* These processes are not felt to be treatable with BCT because of their aggressive nature and high likelihood of failure of local control.

- *Logistics.* Patient preference and autonomy must be respected. In medicine, the ossified model of

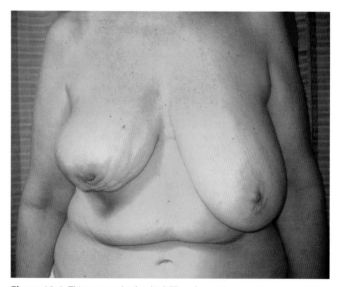

Figure 12.4 This woman had right BCT and over time greater asymmetries have developed. A recurrence was discovered warranting right mastectomy.

paternalism is giving way to joint decision making. Some patients will have sound reasons to prefer BCT or mastectomy, and even when the reasons do not appear so sound to the physicians involved, the competent patient must be the master of her course. Socioeconomic situations including lack of resources to travel to a radiation center, inability to get transportation, and/or competing obligations may lead a woman to choose mastectomy rather than BCT. Interestingly, inability to tolerate lying on a radiation table due to arthritis, injury, or spinal deformities (e.g., kyphoscoliosis) may similarly make a patient a non-candidate for BCT.

- *Collagen vascular disorders.* Active scleroderma or lupus creates concerns for adverse skin and soft tissue toxicity if irradiated. Typically, such a patient should be excluded from BCT and offered mastectomy for disease management. The patient with rheumatoid arthritis is not a contraindication.

- *BRCA status.* Women from strong familial disease lines and/or those tested positive for the BRCA genes should be counseled regarding risk-reducing strategies. If they will consider a contralateral prophylactic mastectomy at some point in the future, it may not be appropriate to receive BCT and accept the side effects of XRT only to have the breast removed in the future. This remains a controversial topic and studies about the efficacy of BCT in women with germline mutations in BRCA 1 or BRCA 2 are equivocal because, although in-breast recurrence is unlikely, new spontaneous tumors in the same or contralateral breast are likely.

- *Pregnancy.* Radiation is to be avoided in the gravid woman because of the significant risks to the developing embryo, which has a low tolerance to the mutagenic effects of radiation, despite the radiation scatter being expected to be low. The risks of radiation-induced malignancy are increased in the fetus exposed to intrauterine radiation.
  - *Caveat.* Nonetheless, if the mother is far enough along in the gestation that she can have a lumpectomy and nodal dissection and commence radiotherapy post partum, it may be feasible to offer BCT + XRT to a pregnant patient. Data indicate that starting radiotherapy up to 10 weeks post surgery is still effective at local control.

- *Multicentric disease.* When two or more separate foci are present, then this may represent a challenge for resecting the lesions without unacceptably deforming the breast or leading to a high-proportion excision of a small-volume breast.
  - *Caveat.* However, if all the tumor(s) are in the same quadrant and are resectable through the same incision with negative margins, then BCT may be offered.

- *Large breasts.* Radiation oncologists have maintained that large pendulous breasts are not suitable for radiation because of the great inhomogeneity in dosage, inconsistent positioning because of skin variability and motion, and poor penetrance through the parenchyma. Furthermore, the large contralateral breast may actually interfere in the beam angles and approaches to deliver radiation to the involved breast. Often these women have been steered towards mastectomy. Figure 12.2 represents a patient who is not an ideal candidate for BCT.
  - *Caveat.* However, bearing in mind oncoplastic principles, these women might be converted into candidates if tumorectomy can be performed through a breast reduction pattern and a contralateral symmetry reduction performed concomitantly. When a breast reduction pattern is utilized, as described elsewhere in this book, one must adhere to oncologic principles of leaving radio-opaque clips in the tumor bed, individualizing the resection pattern to ensure tumor removal, choosing an appropriate flap pedicle to ensure vascularity of the remaining parenchymal tissues, and obtaining a preoperative contralateral screening mammogram. Additional oncoplastic concepts include centralizing the nipple–areola complex, closing the glandular defect by undermining the skin, opposite breast shaping, use of incisions along the junction of aesthetic units such as in the inframammary crease, periareolar region, or the breast meridian.

Predictors of recurrence

The goal of BCT + XRT is to control the risk of local recurrence of breast carcinoma. While late recurrences may occur, 75% of recurrences will occur within 5 years. Late local recurrence has been reported even decades after original BCT. Radiation is a local therapy, and does not provide systemic control, only local control. Certain features of the original tumor enhance the risk of recurrence.

- *Multifocal disease.* Cancer encompassing more than one quadrant of the breast does increase the risk of recurrence. However, it is not an absolute contraindication.

- *Lymphovascular invasion.* Histologically, lymphovascular invasion indicates a tumor biology which is at higher risk for recurrence.

- *Positive or close margin.* The role for radiation as adjuvant therapy is to control recurrence once all detectable disease is excised. Hence, a positive margin should be surgically addressed whenever feasible. A close margin should be considered for further excision if this can be accomplished surgically without distortion of the breast.

- *Extensive intraductal component.* This may be a marker for in-duct spread of tumor and, so long as margins are negative, EIS is not an absolute contraindication for BCT. It does place the patient at higher risk for local failure.

Factors that are not predictors of recurrence include estrogen receptor status, histologic grade, nodal status, and HER2/neu expression. Women with BRCA 1 or BRCA 2 are not at high risk for local in-breast recurrence, so long as they are otherwise good candidates for BCT. However, those preferring a contralateral prophylactic mastectomy as a risk reduction strategy would be better served with a mastectomy. **Figure 12.5** depicts the same patient as in Figure 12.1, who had a good outcome with left BCT and now does have a recurrence. Although not BRCA positive by testing but with a not insignificant family history of cancer, she elected for right prophylactic mastectomy and left mastectomy for recurrent disease. Interestingly, the previously radiated side did not need a mastopexy because of skin tightening from radiation, but the right prophylactic side did need a vertical pattern mastopexy.

Post-mastectomy radiation therapy

Indications

A survival benefit is conferred by administering radiation to those women undergoing a mastectomy who have greater than three lymph node involvement. There is significant survival benefit and local control benefit conferred by PMRT for advanced disease. The criteria are being broadened, emboldened by the increasing safety of radiation therapy, and in certain situations PMRT is utilized in women with only one to three positive axillary nodes. A survival benefit is shown from the EBCTCG meta-analysis data, and the fields of radiation should include chest wall, supraclavicular, and internal mammary nodes. There are increasing data to suggest that internal

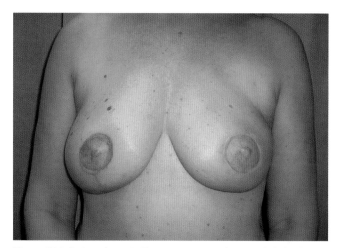

Figure 12.5 Patient shown in Figure 12.1 now undergoes a left therapeutic mastectomy, right prophylactic mastectomy, and bilateral immediate free DIEP flap reconstruction.

mammary lymph node irradiation is important in those with clinically negative axillae, and even more so in those with clinically positive axillae, although some practitioners include the internal mammary nodes only for medial tumors.

Contraindications

Certain overall patient characteristics make them unsuitable for PMRT.

- *Prior radiation.* Exceeding the total allowable dose can create injurious results such as osteoradionecrosis, ulceration, rib fractures, and secondary malignancies.
- *Patient unwillingness.* Even when evidence-based guidelines indicate an absolute survival benefit associated with PMRT, a patient may decline treatment for a variety of factors, rational or irrational. Some patients have great fear about radiation and its effects on the lung or heart, its ability to induce secondary tumors, and its potential effects on the cosmesis of the reconstruction. The patient and her family have to assess their risk aversion in the context of the data available as it applies to their particular scenario.
- *Collagen vascular disorders.* The patient with active lupus or scleroderma is susceptible to accelerated damage from radiation and should be extensively counseled regarding the role of radiation in the overall management of the breast cancer.
- *Pregnancy.* As previously discussed for BCT, post-mastectomy radiation can be initiated up to 10 weeks after surgery with equal efficaciousness. It should not be delivered until the patient is post partum.

Treatment modalities

Over the last 20 years, dramatic improvements in technique and technology have delivered better oncologic endpoints and outcomes. While in BCT whole breast irradiation is the norm, there are some other alternatives that are being trialed and gaining acceptance. Partial breast irradiation (PBI) and accelerated partial breast irradiation (APBI) are being advanced as a way to minimize the 5- to 7-week commitment of the patient to the radiation center, while delivering a biologically effective dose. They deliver radiation into the tumor bed and immediate surrounding tissues, since this is the at-risk zone for tumor reappearance.

PBI methods may be teletherapy or brachytherapy. PBI may be 5 days of twice daily for 15 once-daily fractions, depending on the modality.

Teletherapy

- *Intraoperative tele-radiation therapy.* At the time of lumpectomy, the patient can be treated with a single large fraction of radiation via photons or electrons prior to wound closure. Intraoperative RT has been reported on with 4-year follow-up with no major side effects and an in-field recurrence rate of 0.5%, from the European Institute of Oncology. It was reported in a retrospective study of 355 patients who were not suitable candidates for traditional postoperative XRT and were treated instead with the use of full-dose intraoperative radiotherapy with electrons (ELIOT) in advance of long-term results of ongoing clinical trials, as the sole radiotherapy for patients with unifocal invasive carcinoma who were candidates for BCT. The typical dose was 21 Gy intraoperatively, biologically equivalent to 58–60 Gy in standard fractionation.

ELIOT may be an emerging option for those women who cannot tolerate traditional fractions because of increased susceptibility of their skin, subcutaneous tissue, and contralateral breast and lung from pre-existing morbidities.

- *Postoperative tele-radiation therapy*
  - *Intensity-modulated radiation therapy* (IMRT) has shown improved dose homogeneity and local control equivalent to traditional therapy in the setting of BCT. Static multileaf collimator (sMLC) IMRT technique has been reported in a trial of 281 patients where 56% experienced Radiation Therapy Oncology Group Grade 0 or I acute skin toxicity; 43% developed Grade II acute skin toxicity and only 1% experienced Grade III toxicity. The cosmetic results at 12 months were excellent/good in 99% of the patients. No skin telangiectasias, significant fibrosis, or persistent breast pain was noted. This greater uniformity helps with potential reduction in acute and chronic toxicities while maintaining the efficacy of breast irradiation.
  - *3D conformal methods* show promising results in Phase I and II trials. The planned target volume is the tumor bed plus a 1–2 cm margin defined at post-mastectomy CT. A regimen of five fractions over 10 days is typically performed with total dose range of 25–30 Gy. Cosmesis and tumor control results appear encouraging from early reports.

Brachytherapy

- *Interstitial brachytherapy.* Hollow catheters are inserted through the parenchyma at the time of the lumpectomy, and after simulation these are loaded with a radioactive source, usually iridium-192, via a remote loader. Currently in Phase I/II protocol at Tufts, dose was prescribed to the tumor bed plus a 2 cm margin and a total of 3400 cGy was delivered in 10 fractions twice daily over 5 days. Toxicities (skin, subcutaneous tissue, pain, fat necrosis) were evaluated by Radiation Therapy Oncology Group criteria; cosmesis was assessed using a previously published scale. The actuarial local recurrence rate was 6.1% at 5 years. Fat necrosis was not seen in the first 6 months after treatment, and then plateaued at 18%. Moderate to severe subcutaneous toxicity was seen in 35.7% of patients. The percentage of patients with less than excellent cosmetic outcomes was about 20%. Other trials have used cesium-137 as the radioactive seed instead of iridium-192.

- *Intracavitary brachytherapy.* An example is Mammosite (Cytyc Corporation, Marlborough, MA) whereby a double-lumen balloon catheter is placed at the time of surgery. For a period of 5 days, a computer-controlled high-dose rate HDR machine inserts a radiation 'seed' (iridium-192) to deliver the brachytherapy, and the seed is withdrawn between treatments. On the fifth day, the balloon is removed through the same incision.

A recent study from Rush Medical Center of 70 patients with at least 6 months follow-up showed a crude failure rate of about 7%. Another study reported on 5-year results of 70 prospective enrollees, of whom only 43 patients completed accelerated partial breast irradiation with Mammosite brachytherapy. A dose of 34 Gy was delivered in 10 fractions over 5 days. In some patients cavity size was not amenable to balloon placement or for skin spacing. The infection rate was 9.3% and the seroma rate 32.6%. Good–excellent cosmetic outcomes were achieved in 83.3% of the 36 patients with more than 5 years of follow-up. There were two serious infections. No contralateral cancers developed.

In a subsequent report with 1400 patients, breast seromas were reported in 23.9% of cases (symptomatic in 10.6% of cases), and 1.5% of cases developed fat necrosis. With a median follow-up of 37.5 months, the 3-year actuarial rate of in-breast tumor recurrence was 1.79%.

These early reports highlight the importance of proper patient selection for this evolving technique.

Timing and types of reconstruction

Breast reconstruction is a challenging art because the reconstruction must simultaneously be sensual, soft, a commensurate size to the patient, and symmetric with the opposite breast in unilateral cases. These goals are routinely realizable by tailoring the method to the patient's lifestyle, preferences, and donor site availability. The two broad categories of reconstruction are autologous or implant based. Both of these become yet more nuanced once radiation – either previous or anticipated – enters the picture.

Operating on radiated structures is predictably unpredictable. We can anticipate longer time to ultimate healing, beyond the usual 6 weeks, since every step of the healing cascade is retarded. Flap undermining should be limited since the conventional length:width ratios will be altered. The skin and underlying musculofascial layers are typically woodier, indurated, and have diminution of their viscoelastic properties such as stress relaxation and creep. Telangiectasias, even if not appreciated on the skin prior to incision, will become manifest, and prolonged erythema may present, often confused and treated as cellulitis. There will be variable degrees of fat necrosis in undermined and elevated tissues as well. Because of great variability in patient response to radiation, while these changes can be foreseen, the magnitude of the changes is not predictable, hence caution is advised.

Unfortunately, the aesthetic results are variable as well. Radiated tissue, because it will not be as pliant as non-radiated tissue, throws plans and predictions out of the well-worn grooves of plastic surgery. For instance, in a typical breast reduction the plastic surgeon would anticipate and compensate for 'bottoming-out' and for scars and shape to 'settle-out'. In a post-radiation breast reduction, 'bottoming-out' occurs to a much lesser degree and the aesthetic result of a unilateral breast reduction can be quite stellar. However, the non-radiated breast will experience 'settling-out', thus creating ongoing asymmetry since the two breasts will take dramatically different healing trajectories and paths. **Figure 12.6** demonstrates a patient with a bilateral reduction and their different healing patterns, and is the same patient shown in Figure 12.2. This experience is further amplified in vertical pattern mastopexies and reductions because the subtle challenges of this relatively novel technique are further exacerbated.

So challenging can be the sequelae of radiation injury that sometimes an appropriate method is to 're-create the defect'. Research from Institut Curie in Paris, France, indicated that for unacceptable cosmetic outcomes in up to 5% of their patients, they would perform a completion

mastectomy and immediate reconstruction for a hostile BCT outcome.

There is no consensus on how long to wait after the conclusion of radiotherapy before attempting an operation. Certainly one should wait until the visible signs of injury such as induration and edema are abating. The timeline has to be tailored to the patient and operation may be performed anywhere from 3 months post XRT to 12–24 months post XRT. This may frustrate the patient's calendar since patients are keen to complete their care.

Whenever feasible, immediate reconstruction delivers a superior cosmetic outcome to delayed reconstruction because the full potential of a skin-sparing mastectomy can be exploited in the reconstruction, independent of whether or not there will be or has been radiation. There will likely be a single scar when immediate reconstruction is used with tissue expanders or with autologous flap reconstruction, whereas in delayed reconstruction using flaps a large patch of skin is added creating more than one visible scar. Whenever possible, these additional scars are placed at the junction of aesthetic units such as periareolar or in the inframammary crease.

The two categories of reconstruction methodologies employed are implants and flaps.

Expander/implant reconstruction

Prior radiation

In the patient who has had a past attempt at BCT and had lumpectomy + XRT, the radiation injury will confound attempts at reconstruction when the patient has a recurrence. The well-established dogma in plastic surgery is that implant-based reconstruction in a previously irradiated chest is going to have a higher complication rate. The incidence of infection will be elevated, as will the incidence of capsular contracture, erosion/exposure of the implant, pain, and asymmetry. **Figures 12.7** and **12.8** show a patient with an initial good outcome with implant reconstruction and PMRT, and then loss of the implant on the left due to infection. **Figure 12.9** shows a patient with severe capsular contracture, and is the same patient shown preoperatively in Figure 12.3 with unilateral lymphedema.

There is immense variability in how patients respond to radiotherapy, and that coupled with the specifics of their mastectomy – such as how thick the skin flaps are, how close the tumor was to the skin, if the patient has other co-morbidities such as diabetes or smoking – will impact on the success or failure of the reconstruction.

Skin margin viability must be assiduously checked because it is notoriously difficult to ascertain from gross inspection. Some surgeons use fluorescein and a Wood's lamp to check perfusion, while others rely on clinical inspection. The pectoralis major muscle may have become atrophic and/or woody and firm from the radiation, and may not mobilize without tearing, and will probably lack the pliability that it ordinarily has. Lower initial volumes

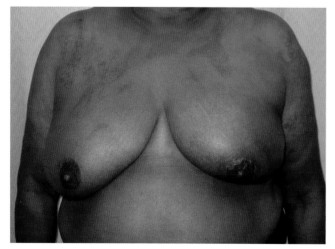

Figure 12.6 Patient shown in Figure 12.2 underwent bilateral breast reduction. The left side pedicle design was modified because of her history of radiation and lumpectomy.

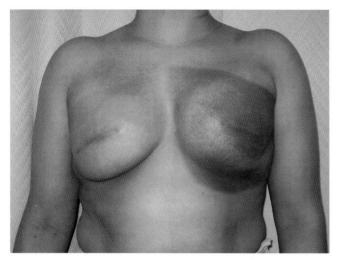

Figure 12.7 This patient underwent left modified radical mastectomy and radiation therapy with implant placement as well as right prophylactic mastectomy and implant placement. Left-sided hyperpigmentation is visible, but no capsular contracture.

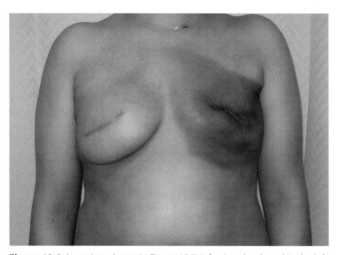

Figure 12.8 In patient shown in Figure 12.7, infection developed in the left breast requiring removal of implant. Implants have higher complication rates in the setting of radiation.

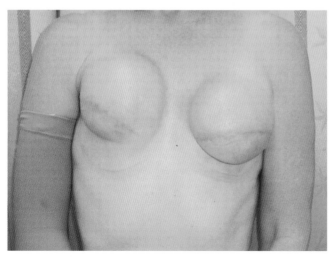

Figure 12.9 Patient shown in Figure 12.3 elected for bilateral implant based reconstruction. Note the right-sided capsular contracture in the setting of prior radiation.

may be placed in the tissue expander, and in-office serial expansions will likely be lower volume and more numerous than in a non-radiated setting.

Planned radiation

Those patients who, based on tumor size, margins, and lymph node status, will proceed with PMRT should be informed that the results obtained with implant-based reconstruction will have limitations in this scenario. Oncoplastic principles dictate that the plastic reconstruction should not delay adjuvant treatments such as chemotherapy and radiotherapy. Hence, the patient will likely proceed with oncologic treatment before she is at full or target expansion. The plan can be placed 'on hold' until those oncologically indicated therapies are complete and the patient has had time to recover. Most expanders have a ferromagnetic integrated port, and so they are not MRI compatible. Any magnetic resonance imaging work-up for the contralateral breast or other body parts should be completed prior to placement of the expander. They do not cause any impediment to radiation therapy, however, since the scatter from the port is clinically insignificant. Rarely, an expander shape interferes with the required vectors to complete radiation planning. In those situations, the expander can be deflated until radiotherapy is completed, and then re-expanded prior to definitive surgery.

Managing complications

The higher incidence of capsular contracture in this situation may have to be managed with over-expansion to retard the constricting effects of the capsule, or with capsulectomies when the expander is exchanged for a permanent implant. There will likely be 'step-offs' where the radiated skin will tend to 'shrink-wrap' down to the underlying chest wall contours, creating a sharp demarcation with the implant in the upper outer pole of the breast. These contour irregularities may be corrected with a biomaterial such as Alloderm acellular human dermis (LifeCell, Branchburg, NJ) or by fat grafts. While autologous fat grafting is gaining acceptance, it remains rife with controversy because of the concerns of fat necrosis causing confusing calcifications in the breast. Local flaps such as a thoracodorsal perforator (TDAP) flap, lateral thoracic flap, or intercostal perforator flaps can be used to recruit vascularized tissue into the defects and ameliorate contour irregularities.

If unyielding complications are present, then the patient may need to be converted to autologous reconstruction.

Autologous flap reconstruction

Prior radiation

If the patient has had prior radiation for an attempt at BCT in the past, reconstruction with autologous tissue, whenever possible, offers the greatest likelihood of a favorable outcome. Because healthy, well-perfused tissue can be brought into a radiated field, it is likely to heal better and support the radiated tissue. A latissimus dorsi musculocutaneous flap or a thoracodorsal artery perforator flap (based on the same vascularity as the latissimus flap, but sparing the muscle) can utilize some of the tissue laxity along the back. However, one must plan to inspect the source vessels since the patient with a prior mastectomy and/or axillary dissection may no longer have patent thoracodorsal vessels. Secondary retrograde perfusion of the flap from collateral flow from the serratus branch may allow latissimus and TDAP flaps to be used even when the primary pedicle is no longer patent.

Similarly, if a pedicled TRAM flap is performed from the abdomen, it is preferable to base it off the contralateral non-irradiated superior epigastric vessels so that it is not reliant on an irradiated pedicle. In the setting of a free flap (free TRAM, free deep inferior epigastric perforator flap, or free gluteal artery perforator flap) even previously irradiated internal mammary vessels or previously irradiated thoracodorsal vessels are usually sufficient. However, prior radiation does make the dissection more demanding, the vessels slightly more friable, and the success rate of free tissue transfer can be 2–4% lower than when non-irradiated vessels are used. A successful reconstruction, nonetheless, is likely and a skin-sparing mastectomy with immediate free flap reconstruction is demonstrated in **Figure 12.10** and is the same patient demonstrated preoperatively in Figure 12.4.

Planned radiation

When autologous tissue reconstruction is planned and the likelihood of the patient receiving PMRT exists (e.g., for multi-node positivity), one can consider either placing a larger flap to accommodate for future atrophy, or place an expander with planned replacement with flap after completion of XRT. Evidence from the MD Anderson experience indicates that, of those who underwent immediate autologous reconstruction, 24% required an additional flap to correct flap contracture and 22% maintained a normal breast volume. Hyperpigmentation occurred in 37% percent of the patients, 56% were noted to have a firm reconstruction, and loss of symmetry ensued in 78%. The findings were statistically significant when compared with 1443 non-irradiated TRAM patients. At our institution, we most frequently consider a 'delayed–immediate' strategy of placing an expander for the duration of the radiation and then, 3–6 months after the conclusion of radiotherapy, removing the expander and performing autologous reconstruction to circumvent the unpredictable volume, contour, and symmetry loss associated with irradiation of flap reconstruction.

Interestingly, at this stage about 15% of our patients will elect to convert the expander to an implant instead of proceeding with a lengthy surgery to perform autologous reconstruction. While the patients are educated about the higher rate of complications in implant-based reconstruction in a radiated bed, they often have favorable outcomes. The remaining 85% do progress to autologous flap reconstruction, and the patient is then treated as someone who has had 'prior radiation'. In **Figure 12.11** is shown a woman who declined 'delayed–immediate' and underwent a mastectomy and PMRT followed by delayed reconstruction. After her reconstruction (**Fig. 12.12**) the flap is warm, soft, and has no fat necrosis, while the surrounding skin remains indurated and telangiectatic. The result is still superior to an immediate flap followed by radiation, but not as good as having an interval 'space-saving' expander during PMRT.

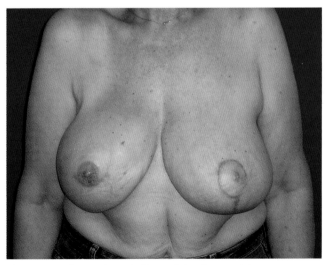

Figure 12.10 Patient shown in Figure 12.4 underwent right mastectomy with oncoplastic principles to spare the skin envelope and reconstruction with a free DIEP flap. The left breast underwent a reduction for symmetry.

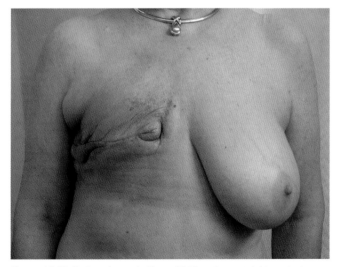

Figure 12.11 Patient shown in Figure 12.10 underwent right mastectomy and received post-mastectomy radiation. She developed unusual skin toxicity from the treatment.

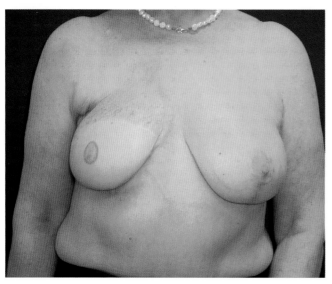

Figure 12.12 Patient shown in Figure 12.11 underwent delayed reconstruction with a free flap to the internal mammary artery and vein, fat grafting to the upper pole and contralateral breast reduction.

Managing complications

Complications of autologous reconstruction are most often related to partial or complete loss of the transported tissues. If this happens, local tissue rearrangement may correct the problem. In instances of total flap loss, a second flap (most often a free flap) will have to be recruited once the underlying cause of flap failure has been understood and resolved. In the instance of free tissue transfer, alternative donor vessels such as thoracodorsal, internal mammaries, contralateral mammary vessels, or thoracoacromials may have to be dissected.

Reconstruction options for partial defects are very similar to reconstruction of full defects. Occasionally patients with a lumpectomy defect will wish to camouflage that defect with a small implant. This is possible, but it changes the shape of the breast. Often one has to place an implant in the contralateral breast as well to achieve a similar shape and size. The implants will have to be of different volumes to account for both the volume resected during lumpectomy and the volume of atrophic loss from the secondary effects of XRT.

Alternatively, a woman could select for autologous repair of a BCT defect. Because the reconstructive effort should be proportionate to the defect, a woman may not want the drawbacks of both lumpectomy + XRT and reconstruction. However, if the outcome after BCT is not cosmetically acceptable, then reconstruction of the partial defect is warranted. Local flaps would include an intercostal perforator flap, TDAP flap, lateral thoracic flap, latissimus flap, TRAM flap, or free TRAM or DIEP flap, depending on the magnitude of the defect. Rarely, a completion mastectomy may be warranted if the outcome of BCT is poor enough and a complete autologous reconstruction undertaken.

An interesting socioeconomic challenge faced by breast cancer survivors seeking repair of BCT defects is the possibility that it may not be covered by their insurance company. The Women's Health and Cancer Rights Act of 1998 (WHCRA) is a federal mandate obligating coverage of benefits for breast reconstruction after mastectomy and symmetry operations on the normal breast. It does not apply to a woman who has had BCT, although broadly third-party payers have covered plastic surgical reconstruction of BCT related defects.

Summary

Breast cancer is a common disease that is being approached in a multidisciplinary fashion via a concerted effort of medical oncologists, radiation oncologists, surgical oncologists, and plastic surgeons to yield progress in patient care.

The adjuvant use of radiation has been a game-changer in the management of breast cancer and has created the ability to offer breast conservation therapy, which is equi-efficacious to mastectomy in terms of local recurrence and overall survival. Advances in the delivery of radiation include accelerated treatments and partial breast irradiation techniques, which are in their ascendancy.

Some of the challenges created by breast conservation approaches are how to manage the recurrence requiring mastectomy in a previously radiated field or how to solve the cosmetic limitations and complications that might arise from lumpectomy and radiation. Plastic surgery is able to rise to this challenge via implant-based reconstructions or autologous vascularized flaps to repair the defects.

Further reading

Intra M, Leonardi C, Luini A, et al. Full-dose intraoperative radiotherapy with electrons in breast surgery: broadening the indications. Arch Surg 2005; 140(10):936–939.

Veronesi U, Orecchia R, Luini A, et al. Full-dose intraoperative radiotherapy with electrons during breast-conserving surgery: experience with 590 cases. Ann Surg 2005; 242(1):101–106.

Veronesi U, Gatti G, Luini A, et al. Full-dose intraoperative radiotherapy with electrons during breast-conserving surgery. Arch Surg 2003; 138(11): 1253–1256.

Clough KB, Thomas SS, Fitoussi AD, et al. Reconstruction after conservative treatment for breast cancer: cosmetic sequelae classification revisited. Plast Reconstr Surg 2004; 114(7):1743–1753.

Clough KB, Cuminet J, Fitoussi A, et al. Cosmetic sequelae after conservative treatment for breast cancer: classification and results of surgical correction. Ann Plast Surg 1998; 41(5):471–481.

Clough KB, Kroll SS, Audretsch W. An approach to the repair of partial mastectomy defects. Plast Reconstr Surg 1999; 104(2):409–420.

Fisher B, Redmond C, Fisher ER, et al. Ten-year results of a randomized clinical trial comparing radical mastectomy and total mastectomy with or without radiation. N Engl J Med 1985; 312(11):674–681.

Tran NV, Evans GR, Kroll SS, et al. Postoperative adjuvant irradiation: effects on transverse rectus abdominis muscle flap breast reconstruction. Plast Reconstr Surg 2000; 106(2):313–317; discussion 318–320.

Kronowitz SJ, Hunt KK, Kuerer HM, et al. Practical guidelines for repair of partial mastectomy defects using the breast reduction technique in patients undergoing breast conservation therapy. Plast Reconstr Surg 2007; 120(7):1755–1768.

Kronowitz SJ, Hunt KK, Kuerer HM, et al. Delayed-immediate breast reconstruction. Plast Reconstr Surg 2004; 113(6):1617–1628.

Asgeirsson KS, Rasheed T, McCulley SJ, et al. Oncological and cosmetic outcomes of oncoplastic breast conserving surgery. Eur J Surg Oncol 2005; 31(8):817–823.

Formenti SC, Rosenstein B, Skinner KA, et al. T1 stage breast cancer: adjuvant hypofractionated conformal radiation therapy to tumor bed in selected postmenopausal breast cancer patients: pilot feasibility study. Radiology 2002; 222(1):171–178.

Vicini FA, Sharpe M, Kestin L, et al. Optimizing breast cancer treatment efficacy with intensity-modulated radiotherapy. Int J Radiat Oncol Biol Phys 2002; 54(5):1336–1344.

Clough KB, Lewis JS, Couturaud B, et al. Oncoplastic techniques allow extensive resections for breast-conserving therapy of breast carcinomas. Ann Surg 2003; 237(1):26–34.

Swanson TA, Vicini FA. Overview of accelerated partial breast irradiation. Curr Oncol Rep 2008; 10(1):54–60.

Vicini F, Beitsch PD, Quiet CA, et al. Three-year analysis of treatment efficacy, cosmesis, and toxicity by the American Society of Breast Surgeons MammoSite Breast Brachytherapy Registry Trial in patients treated with accelerated partial breast irradiation (APBI). Cancer 2008; 112(4):758–766.

Benitez PR, Keisch ME, Vicini F, et al. Five-year results: the initial clinical trial of MammoSite balloon brachytherapy for partial breast irradiation in early-stage breast cancer. Am J Surg 2007; 194(4):456–462.

Bovi J, Qi XS, White J, et al. Comparison of three accelerated partial breast irradiation techniques: treatment effectiveness based upon biological models. Radiother Oncol 2007; 84(3):226–232.

Kaufman SA, DiPetrillo TA, Price LL, et al. Long-term outcome and toxicity in a Phase I/II trial using high-dose-rate multicatheter interstitial brachytherapy for T1/T2 breast cancer. Brachytherapy 2007; 6(4):286–292.

Spear SL, Onyewu C. Staged breast reconstruction with saline-filled implants in the irradiated breast: recent trends and therapeutic implications. Plast Reconstr Surg 2000; 105(3):930–942.

Management of the Contralateral Breast Following Oncoplastic Surgery

Maurice Y Nahabedian • Justin West

Introduction

The management of the contralateral breast following breast conservation therapy (BCT) or oncoplastic surgery is an important yet frequently overlooked component of reconstructive breast surgery. It is now well appreciated that reconstructive breast surgery has improved the quality of life for many women following partial or total removal; however, unless breast symmetry is achieved, patient satisfaction may not be optimized.[1] Although oncoplastic surgery can be successfully performed without a contralateral procedure, it is useful in many women. This is especially true following oncoplastic surgery in which greater amounts of normal breast parenchyma are excised, which will exacerbate any resultant volume or contour asymmetry. Although the exact incidence of these contralateral procedures has not been reported following oncoplastic surgery, it has been reported to range from 15% to 89% following total mastectomy and immediate breast reconstruction.[2,3]

The purpose of this chapter is to review the techniques, concepts, and principles for contralateral breast operations in the setting of oncoplastic breast surgery. The most common techniques include reduction mammaplasty, mastopexy, and augmentation. Many of these essential concepts have been reviewed in the previous chapters; however, this chapter will focus primarily on the contralateral breast and secondarily on the ipsilateral breast because the two are co-dependent.

Indications and contraindications

Contralateral breast procedures will improve breast symmetry in many women following oncoplastic surgery. There are essentially three different contralateral operations that can be performed: a reduction mammaplasty, mastopexy, and augmentation (**Box 13.1**). In the case of volume discrepancy, a reduction mammaplasty may be indicated; in the case of contour discrepancy, a mastopexy may be indicated; and in the reverse case in which the contralateral breast is smaller, an augmentation using a prosthetic device may be indicated. The factors guiding these decisions include patient and breast characteristics, timing of surgery, cancer stage, margin status, and postoperative radiation treatments. The contraindications for contralateral breast operations will be related to patient desire, oncologic risks of developing a contralateral breast cancer, and breast characteristics. These factors will be further reviewed.

Preoperative history and considerations

A number of factors should be considered when counseling patients regarding surgery of the contralateral breast. First, the surgeon should confirm that the patient has been thoroughly evaluated for the presence of cancer in that breast. Next, the surgeon must determine the patients' goals regarding size and shape of the breasts, as well as the position and size of the nipple–areolar complex (NAC). Patients with large breasts should be questioned about associated problems such as back and neck pain, grooving from bra straps, and infections. Risk factors for poor outcomes, such as obesity and tobacco use, should be addressed and appropriately managed. Finally, patients should be educated about the increased risk of breast cancer in the contralateral breast and counseled regarding the importance of continued surveillance by both routine physical exam and breast imaging.

Patient selection

Women who may benefit from a contralateral procedure can be considered in two ways: those who need recontouring and those who need volume adjustments. All of these women have one common denominator: they have all undergone a unilateral oncologic operation and decided to preserve the NAC. The importance of a natural appearance and symmetry should not be underestimated. These women may range in age from young (<30 years of age) to elderly (>65 years of age); however, the majority of women are middle aged, have had children, and have breasts that have become increasingly pendulous, voluminous, and/or ptotic. In some of these women, resection of the primary breast cancer may not result in a perceptible change in contour or volume and obviate the need for a contralateral procedure. However, in other women, a lumpectomy or partial mastectomy can result in a perceptible change and asymmetry between the two breasts. For these women, contralateral operations may be useful.

All women considering oncoplastic surgery are required to undergo imaging studies of both breasts via mammography or magnetic resonance imaging (MRI). The presence of an abnormality in the contralateral breast would be a contraindication for a purely aesthetic operation and would necessitate oncologic evaluation. Women are informed that the cancerous breast following oncoplastic management will be irradiated and should be informed that the breast contour may be altered following the radiation treatments. This fact may influence the decision regarding whether or not to have the contralateral procedure performed immediately or on a delayed basis.

Timing of surgery

The decision to have an immediate or delayed contralateral procedure is dependent upon a variety of factors, which include patient desire, the ability to completely resect the primary tumor, recognition of postoperative and post-radiation changes, and the feasibility of coordinating an operation between the oncologic and reconstructive surgeon. The long-term outcomes are essentially the same, other than the fact that the patient will be asymmetric in the short run. Many women prefer to undergo one procedure, the principal reason being that both breasts can be operated upon at the same time. Prominent volume or contour asymmetries can be a source of dissatisfaction for some women.

An important consideration that influences the timing of the contralateral operation is the ability to completely resect the primary tumor. If the tumor is small and localized and the oncologic surgeon is confident that the tumor has been excised with an acceptable margin of resection, then the acquired deformity can be reconstructed and a contralateral procedure for symmetry performed at the same time. If there are any concerns based on the fact that the tumor is larger than expected, is multifocal, or that an adequate margin of resection is uncertain, then reconstruction of the ipsilateral and contralateral breast should be delayed. Some women may decide to observe the outcome of the initial operation and then decide whether or not to have a contralateral procedure. The advantage of this approach is that margin status can be pathologically confirmed and specific asymmetries noted.

The final consideration is the ability to coordinate schedules between the oncologic and reconstructive surgeons. Obviously, with a delayed contralateral procedure, this will not be a factor; however, in immediate cases, it may. In women with moderate to severe mammary hypertrophy or breast ptosis, a reduction mammaplasty or mastopexy may be needed. Many surgeons support addressing the opposite breast at the time of the cancer surgery because the contralateral breast serves as a model by which the reconstructed breast is patterned. Immediate reduction of the contralateral breast also allows for histological examination of the resected tissues with the potential to find and treat occult disease. On the other hand, some surgeons will endorse a delayed approach, allowing ample time for postsurgical and radiation changes to evolve. Although a secondary procedure may become necessary, proponents will argue that the results are more predictable.

It is an accepted belief that the oncologic portions of the operation are performed by a surgeon specializing in ablative procedures and that the reconstructive portions are performed by a reconstructive specialist. In some settings, the ablative surgeons are comfortable with the reconstructive portions of the operation as well. In these cases coordinating schedules will not be a factor. However, in other situations where the reconstructive portion of the ipsilateral and contralateral breast will be more complicated, a surgeon specializing in breast reconstruction should be involved.

Oncologic considerations

As part of the breast cancer management team, it is important for plastic surgeons to be familiar with the cancer risks women face following treatment of breast cancer. A personal history of breast cancer is the number one risk of developing breast cancer in the contralateral breast.[4,5] It has been reported that women who have had cancer have a 2–5 times higher risk of getting a cancer in the contralateral breast compared to other women.[6–8] Other studies have suggested that the risk of developing a new cancer is about 0.5–1% per year.[9,10] Up to 5–10% of patients with a primary breast cancer will get a contralateral breast cancer sometime in their lifetime.[6,9,11,12]

After breast cancer treatment, women are advised to continue with breast cancer surveillance via physical examination and breast imaging. Women who have had surgery on the contralateral breast for symmetry are advised to obtain a new baseline mammogram 6 months following the operation. Mammographic and clinical findings should be considered more suspicious than in patients without breast cancer.[13] Reduction mammaplasty will alter the parenchymal architecture of the breast and result in microcalcifications. However, these findings are no different from changes associated with other breast procedures such as biopsies and lumpectomies. These changes are easily distinguished from suspicious lesions by experienced breast imagers. It has been demonstrated that reduction of the breasts does not interfere with cancer surveillance.[14]

The surgeon should be prepared to answer questions patients have about the risk of operating on the contralateral breast with regard to a new cancer and the detection of breast cancer. Certain symmetry procedures have been reported to facilitate a woman's ability to detect cancer and may be beneficial as a risk reduction maneuver. It has been reported that breast reduction can result in a 28% decrease in the risk of breast cancer.[14] Furthermore, reducing the contralateral breast allows for evaluation of the pathologic status of the breast. In one series occult tumors were identified in 4.5% of contralateral breast reduction specimens in patients undergoing a symmetry procedure for breast reconstruction.[15,16]

There is a smaller subset of patients that are candidates for breast augmentation following BCT or oncoplastic surgery. In general, these are women with relative micromastia who would have considered breast augmentation in the absence of a diagnosis of breast cancer. Patients who consider or have augmentation with prosthetic devices should be counseled about the need for specialized breast screening. When using the standard craniocaudal and medial–lateral–oblique views of screening mammography for women with implants, up to 40% of the breast parenchyma is potentially obscured. For this reason, specialized implant displacement views have been developed.[17] With these views, an implant in the subglandular position obscures 35% of the breast, and the submuscular position obscures 15%. Thus, women should be made aware that the presence of an implant may hinder breast cancer detection.

Operative technique

Surgical anatomy

The blood supply to the breast comes from perforating branches of the internal mammary, lateral thoracic, thoracodorsal, thoracoacromial, and intercostal arteries and veins[18] (**Fig. 13.1**). The sensory innervation of the breast is dermatomal and derived from the anterolateral and anteromedial branches of the thoracic intercostal nerves T2–T6.[19] Sensation to the NAC is principally derived from the fourth thoracic intercostal nerve. When designing and executing any aesthetic operation on the breast, the vascularity and innervation must be considered. Poorly designed operations can result in nipple–areolar necrosis, loss of nipple areolar sensation, delayed healing, fat necrosis, and persistent asymmetry.[20–24] There are several methods by which a given breast can be reduced in volume or altered in shape.

The ensuing sections will review the authors' preferred methods of reduction mammaplasty, mastopexy, and augmentation. The operative techniques that will be reviewed can be performed immediately (at the time of oncoplastic resection) or on a delayed basis. In general, reduction mammaplasty procedures are performed immediately or on a delayed basis, whereas mastopexy and augmentation are always performed on a delayed basis. The specific reduction technique can be a vertical or short scar approach or the traditional 'inverted T' using the Wise pattern. The specific approach is dependent upon the plastic surgeon's preference and level of comfort. In general, the short scar techniques are used for resections less than 300 g and the Wise pattern is used for resections greater than 300 g. Mastopexy is performed with various patterns that include a circumareolar approach, a circumvertical approach, and an inverted T or Wise pattern approach. Breast augmentation is rarely used but may be considered in select cases. The various techniques will be briefly described.

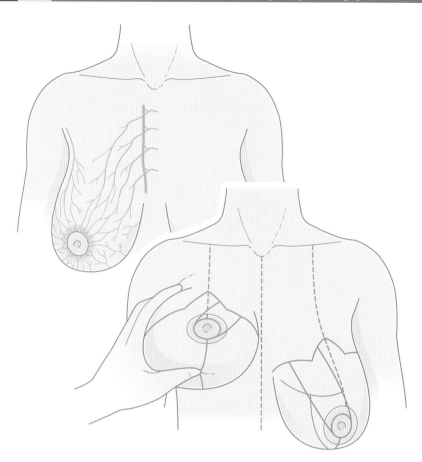

Immediate contralateral reduction mammaplasty using a Wise pattern

Preoperative markings

In patients who will have immediate bilateral reduction mammaplasty following unilateral oncoplastic surgery, several considerations are important. The first is that the specific reduction technique may be different for the two breasts. This is because the specific location of the resected tumor may alter the orientation of the pedicle. The reconstructive surgeon should have a general idea or concept of how the breast will appear following the procedure. The contralateral breast will serve as a template for the oncoplastic breast. Another consideration is that the cancer breast will be radiated and the contralateral breast will not. This may cause the oncoplastic breast to shrink; therefore, that breast should be reconstructed to be slightly larger than the non-cancerous breast.

There are several important landmarks that are delineated prior to the reduction. These include the sternal midline, the inframammary fold, and the breast meridian (**Fig. 13.2**). The breast meridian is determined by marking the mid clavicle and then delineating the midline of the breast. Usually this will bisect the NAC; however, when the NAC is medially or laterally displaced, the meridian will be to the right or left of the NAC (**Fig. 13.3**). The location of the NAC is usually based at the level of the inframammary fold (IMF) at the point where the breast

meridian is bisected. A Wise pattern is delineated on both breasts (**Fig. 13.3**).

The orientation of the pedicle that will ultimately perfuse the NAC is an important consideration. For upper pole tumors, an inferior pedicle is preferred. For lower pole tumors, a superior, superomedial, or medial pedicle is preferred. For medially or laterally based tumors, the pedicle is oriented such that the resulting deformity can be adequately filled. This is usually achieved using a pedicle that is oriented 180 degrees away from the defect.

Technique

The ablative surgeon is advised to proceed with the resection of the tumor. If the tumor is within the delineated Wise pattern then the incision can be placed either on or within the pattern (**Fig. 13.4**). If the tumor is outside the Wise pattern, the incisions may have to be extended in order to facilitate the excision (**Fig. 13.5**). This may alter the appearance of the incisions when comparing the two breasts; however, it is acceptable following maturation of the scars. Following excision of the tumor and surrounding parenchyma, the specimen is weighed and the volume is assessed.

Attention is directed toward the contralateral breast. In general, a medial pedicle is preferred, especially when the anticipated resection volume will exceed 600 g and the NAC requires >6 cm of elevation. A superomedial pedicle is usually preferred when the NAC is elevated more than

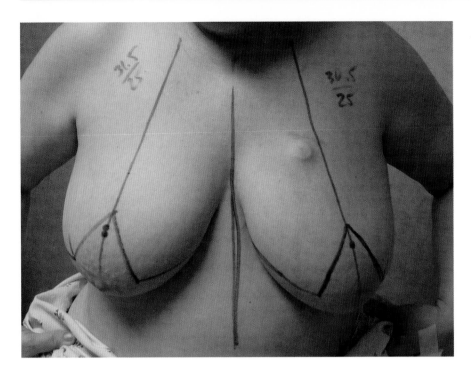

Figure 13.2 Patient photograph demonstrating the breast markings and the Wise pattern. The distance from the sternal notch to the NAC as well as the new nipple position is noted. The breast meridian bisects the NAC.

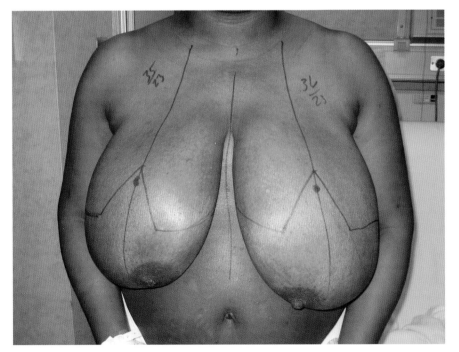

Figure 13.3 A woman with severe macromastia is illustrated. The true breast meridian is delineated lateral to the existing NAC. The final position of the NAC will be along the meridian.

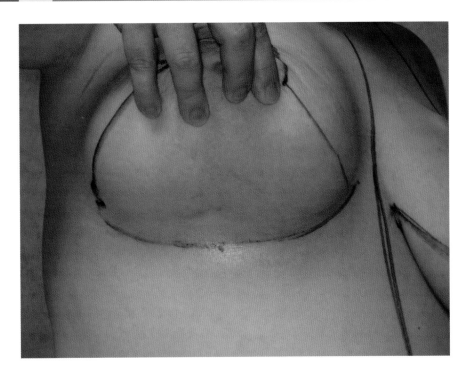

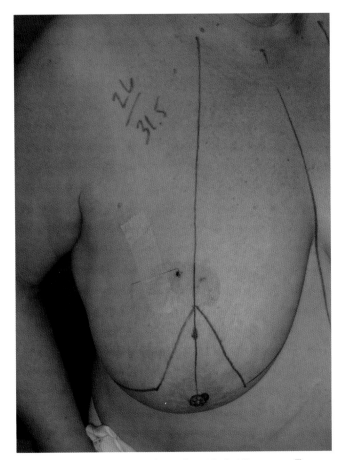

Figure 13.5 The breast tumor is located outside the Wise pattern. The incision will be placed along the upper breast meridian at the site of the tumor.

6 cm. This is because the longer pedicles will rotate on an arc more easily than the shorter pedicles. Short pedicles often require a back-cut along the dermis of the proximal pedicle to facilitate rotation without kinking. An inferior pedicle is used when the length of the nipple to IMF is less than the length of the delineated medial pedicle or when the majority of breast volume is superiorly located.

The first step is to inscribe the NAC with a 38–45 mm cookie cutter (**Fig. 13.6**). The perimeter of the inscription is incised and the pedicle is de-epithelialized (**Fig. 13.7**). The Wise pattern markings are then incised. Dermoglandular wedge excisions are then performed. For a medial or superomedial pedicle, the dermoglandular excision is primarily inferior and lateral (**Fig. 13.8**). For an inferior pedicle, the dermoglandular excision is predominantly superior and lateral. The handling of the vascularized pedicle is important. In general, the pectoral attachments of the pedicle are preserved in order to optimize blood supply. The vascularity of the pedicle and NAC is derived from the subdermal plexus and the intercostal/pectoral perforating vessels (**Fig. 13.9**). Perfusion to the NAC is assessed by adequate arterial bleeding from the dermal edges. Following the dermoglandular excision, the pedicle is rotated toward the apex of the vertical limbs of the Wise pattern (**Fig. 13.10**) and the reduction pattern is closed (**Fig. 13.11**).

At this point the difference in weight is calculated. Usually, the weight of the contralateral specimen is two to three times that of the ipsilateral specimen. Attention is redirected toward the ipsilateral breast and additional

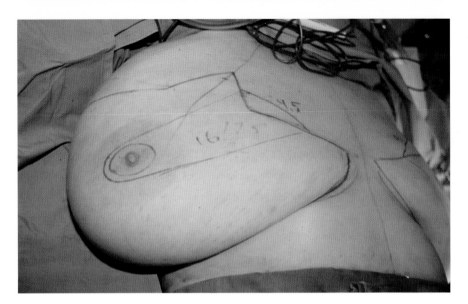

Figure 13.6 The NAC is delineated with a 42 mm diameter and the medial pedicle is drawn as shown.

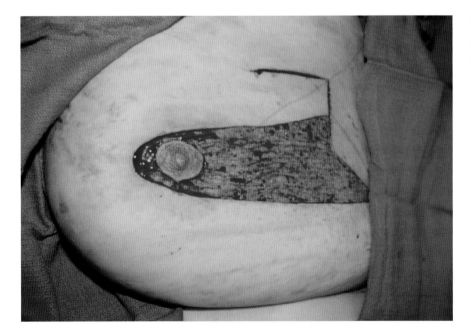

Figure 13.7 The medial pedicle is de-epithelialized. The subdermal plexus of vessels are preserved to improve vascularity to the pedicle and nipple.

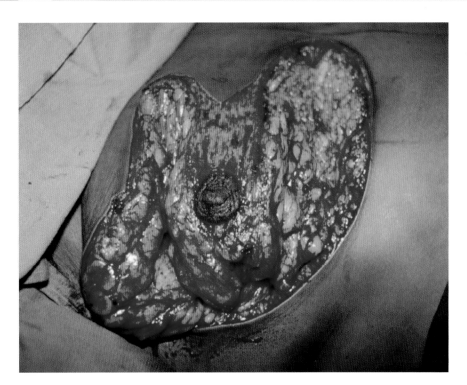

Figure 13.8 The inferior, lateral, medial, and superior dermoglandular wedge excisions are completed, maintaining the medial pedicle.

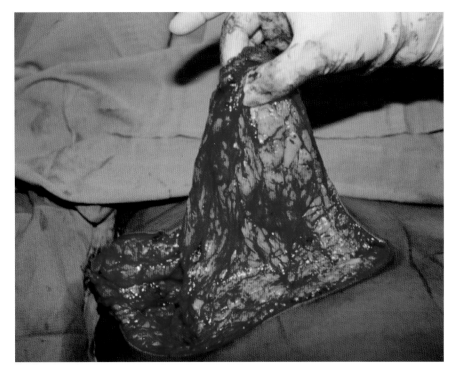

Figure 13.9 The medial pedicle is elevated, demonstrating pectoral muscle attachment for improved vascularity.

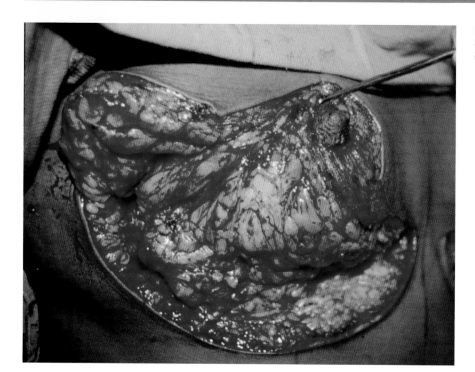

Figure 13.10 The NAC and the medial pedicle are rotated toward the apex of the vertical limbs of the Wise pattern.

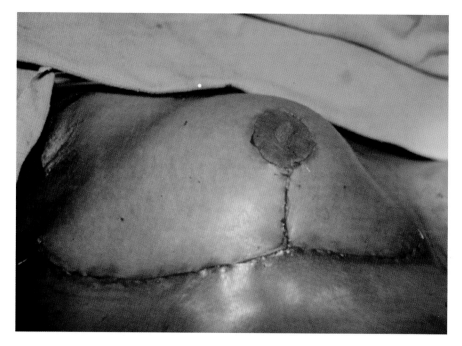

Figure 13.11 The incisions are closed in an inverted T fashion. The position of the NAC is approximately 5 cm from the inframammary fold.

breast parenchyma is resected based upon the location of the primary tumor and the location of excess tissue. In general, it is recommended to leave the ipsilateral breast slightly larger than the contralateral breast to account for the shrinkage that will occur following radiation therapy. The exact amount to leave behind is impossible to quantitate and will depend upon the surgeon's ability to visually assess volume and contour. Once complete, the skin is closed on both breasts. A typical case is illustrated in **Figure 13.12**.

Delayed contralateral reduction mammaplasty following ipsilateral partial mastectomy

In the delayed setting, the markings for a reduction mammaplasty are slightly altered. This is because there is usually a significant breast asymmetry that has occurred. On the cancer side, the location of the NAC is elevated and the breast volume is reduced. The breast has also been previously irradiated. Usually in this situation an ipsilateral reconstructive procedure is needed, such as a latissimus dorsi flap in conjunction with a contralateral breast reduction. To illustrate this concept, a case example will be described in which a partial mastectomy was performed involving the left upper outer quadrant of the breast (**Figs 13.13** and **13.14**). The postoperative radiation resulted in significant displacement of the NAC and breast asymmetry. In this case a latissimus dorsi flap would be used to restore volume, increase the surface area of the cutaneous envelope, and lower the NAC of the ipsilateral breast as well as contralateral reduction mammaplasty to achieve symmetry.

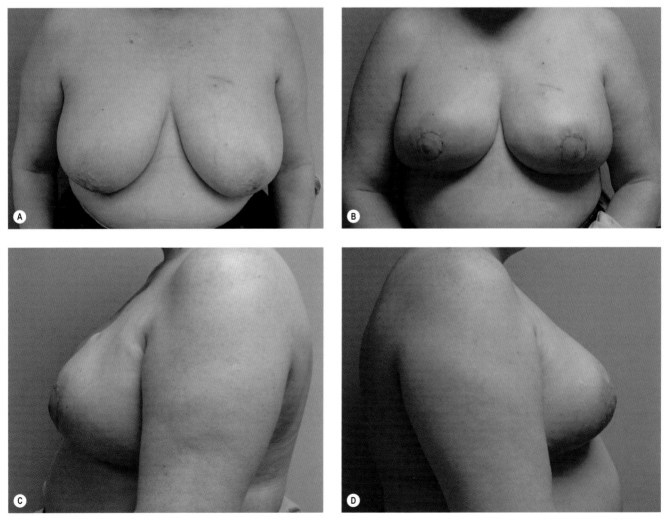

Figure 13.12 (**A**) Preoperative photograph of a woman with left breast cancer who will have oncoplastic surgery and immediate contralateral reduction mammaplasty. (**B**) Postoperative view following left oncoplastic surgery and contralateral reduction mammaplasty. (**C**) Postoperative lateral view of the oncoplastic breast. (**D**) Postoperative lateral view of the contralateral breast following reduction mammaplasty.

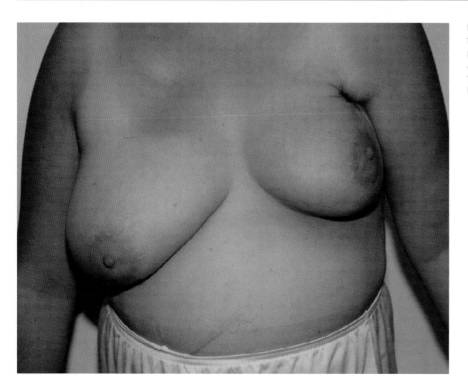

Figure 13.13 Preoperative view of a woman following left partial mastectomy and postoperative irradiation, demonstrating asymmetry and superolateral displacement of the NAC. The plan is to reconstruct the left breast and reduce the contralateral breast.

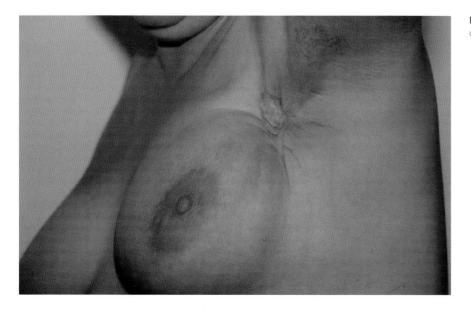

Figure 13.14 Axillary view demonstrating contracture and a cutaneous deficiency.

Preoperative markings

As with the immediate reduction mammaplasty, the IMFs, sternal midline, and breast meridian are delineated (**Fig. 13.15**). The preferred location of the NAC is marked on each breast such that they are on a similar horizontal axis. The NAC is often laterally or superiorly displaced; however, it can also be inferiorly or medially displaced depending on the primary tumor resection site. The goal in these situations is to restore the volume and contour of the ipsilateral breast and to perform a reduction mammaplasty on the contralateral breast. In order to appreciate the amount of reduction needed on the contralateral breast, the ipsilateral deficiency must be first addressed. The distance that the NAC is lowered is determined based upon the location of the nipple on the contralateral breast. As an example, if the ipsilateral NAC is lowered by 5 cm, then at least 5 cm of skin is required on the cutaneous portion of the latissimus dorsi musculocutaneous flap.

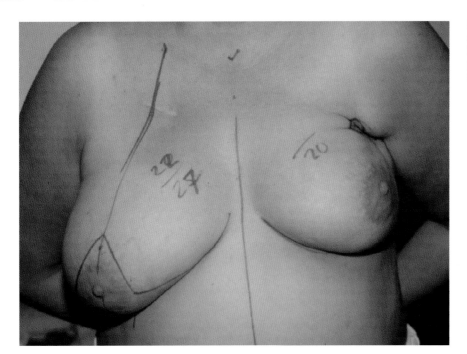

Figure 13.15 Preoperative markings demonstrating the new position of the NAC on both breasts. The breast meridian and Wise pattern have been delineated on the contralateral breast.

Technique

The patient is initially positioned in the lateral decubitus position, on a beanbag, with the ipsilateral breast exposed. The first requirement is to incise the ipsilateral scar and re-create the defect created by the partial mastectomy. Often the size of the defect exceeds what one would generally expect, especially in the setting of postoperative radiation. The dimensions of the cutaneous defect are measured and used to determine the dimensions of the cutaneous component of the latissimus dorsi flap (**Fig. 13.16**). The latissimus dorsi flap is harvested in the standard fashion. The detail of latissimus dorsi flap elevation will not be covered in this section as the emphasis is on the management of the contralateral breast. Once the flap is elevated, it is tunneled into the ipsilateral defect. At this time, the patient is repositioned to the supine position, and re-prepped and draped. The flap is inset and the patient is flexed to 40 degrees to assess breast position and symmetry (**Fig. 13.17**). Adjustments in the contralateral Wise pattern may be necessary to ensure that the NAC is symmetric bilaterally. The details of the reduction mammaplasty are as described in the previous section of this chapter. The final outcome is demonstrated in **Figures 13.18–13.20**.

Delayed bilateral reduction mammaplasty following unilateral oncoplastic surgery

In women with preoperative bilateral mammary hypertrophy, a unilateral oncoplastic operation may still result

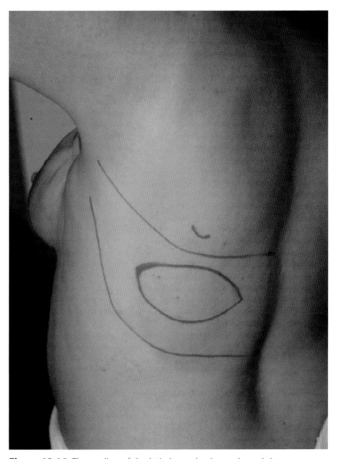

Figure 13.16 The outline of the latissimus dorsi muscle and the cutaneous paddle of the latissimus dorsi musculocutaneous flap have been delineated.

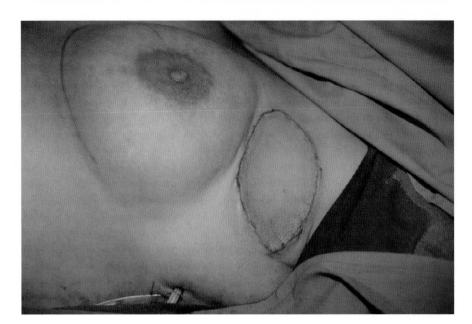

Figure 13.17 Following release of scar tissue in the left breast, the defect is recreated. The latissimus dorsi musculocutaneous flap is harvested and tunneled into the breast defect and inset.

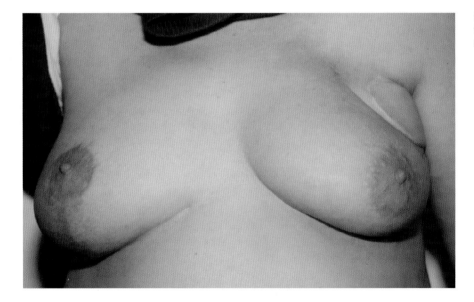

Figure 13.18 Postoperative anterior view following contralateral reduction mammaplasty demonstrating improved symmetry.

in bilateral hypertrophy. Complicating this situation is that there may be both a volume and contour asymmetry in the setting of unilateral radiation therapy. In these situations, some women will be interested in having a bilateral reduction mammaplasty to improve appearance and comfort. To illustrate the complexity of this scenario, a specific case will be described that highlights the features of the operation (**Fig. 13.21**).

Markings and technique

As with the previous markings, the ideal location of the NAC is determined. A reduction pattern is selected and delineated (**Fig. 13.22**). In this case, the partial mastec-

tomy was in the lower quadrant of the left breast and had resulted in superior displacement of the IMF and upper pole fullness. The specific pedicle selected was based on the distance of NAC elevation as well as the site of maximal tissue resection. In this case, a disproportionate amount of tissue was to be excised from the upper pole of the left breast; therefore, an inferior pedicle was selected (**Fig. 13.23**). On the contralateral breast, the plan was to raise the level of the IMF; therefore, a superomedial pedicle was selected.

The salient aspects of the contralateral operation included an elevation of the IMF. This was accomplished by delineating a neo-skin edge along the lower pole of

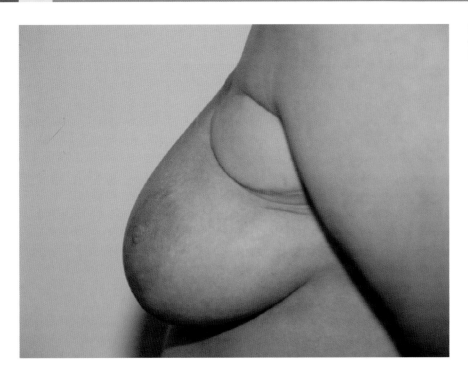

Figure 13.19 Postoperative left lateral view demonstrating final flap position and acceptable breast contour.

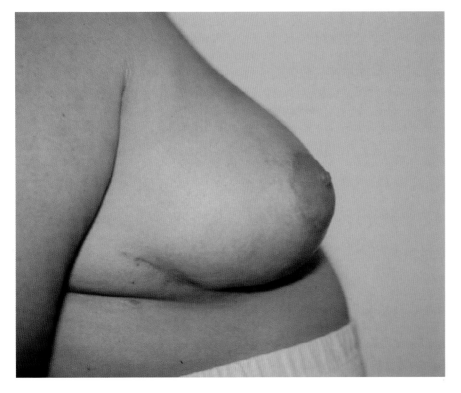

Figure 13.20 Postoperative right lateral view of the contralateral breast, demonstrating ideal positioning of the NAC and acceptable breast contour.

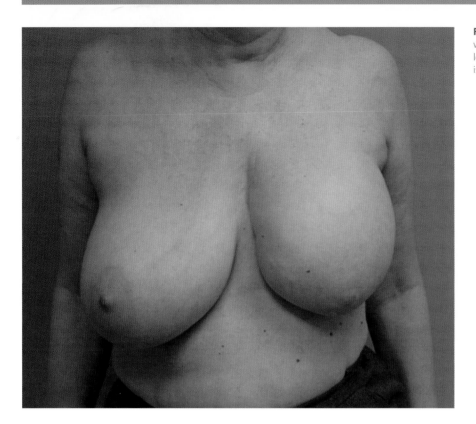

Figure 13.21 Preoperative view of a woman with bilateral mammary hypertrophy following left partial mastectomy and irradiation. The plan is to perform a bilateral reduction mammaplasty.

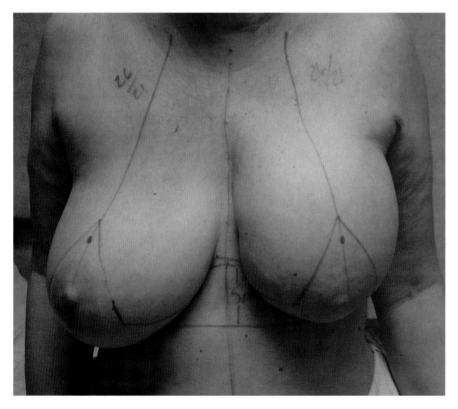

Figure 13.22 The preoperative markings demonstrating equal distance of the sternal notch to nipple distance despite an asymmetry at the level of the inframammary folds and upper pole of the breasts.

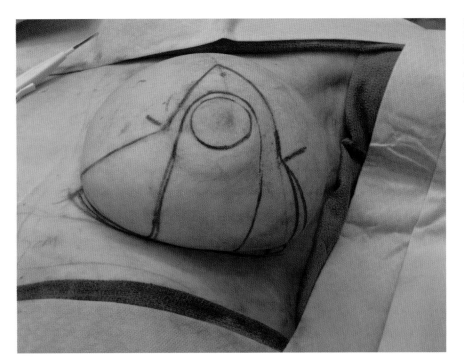

Figure 13.23 The reduction pattern for the left breast will include the Wise pattern with an inferior pedicle technique. The contralateral breast will include a Wise pattern with a central cone technique. The different techniques are selected in order to address the different locations of the tissue to be resected.

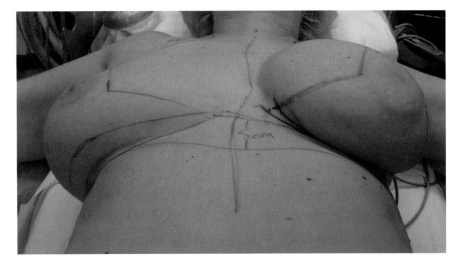

Figure 13.24 A worm's-eye view demonstrating the new position of the inframammary fold on the contralateral breast.

the breast approximately 5 cm above the existing IMF (**Fig. 13.24**). Following resection of the lower pole parenchyma, the lower skin flap was defatted. The dermal edge was sutured at the level of the new IMF using non-absorbable sutures. The ipsilateral breast was managed differently. The NAC was preserved on an inferiorly based dermoparenchymal pedicle with a broad pectoral attachment (**Fig. 13.25**). The upper pole parenchyma was resected while maintaining good perfusion to the skin flaps. An early postoperative photograph demonstrates improved symmetry and contour (**Fig. 13.26**).

Delayed contralateral mastopexy following ipsilateral oncoplastic surgery

Mastopexy of the contralateral breast is indicated when there is contour asymmetry in the presence of volume symmetry. This is often observed following an oncoplastic procedure of the upper breast resulting in superior displacement of the NAC without an appreciable volume loss. Given that postoperative radiation will be performed, it is prudent to delay the contralateral mastopexy in order to assess the degree of modification needed. The effects of radiation following oncoplastic surgery may result in shrinkage or distortion of the ipsilateral breast. The decision as to whether a mastopexy or reduction mammaplasty be performed is best made after all tissue alterations have subsided.

There are several techniques by which a mastopexy may be performed that are based upon the amount of elevation required and degree of breast ptosis. The classification of breast ptosis is provided in Table 13.1. The techniques include the circumareolar, circumvertical, and the inverted T or Wise pattern (**Fig. 13.27**). The circumareolar technique is preferred when less than 2 cm of NAC elevation is required. The circumvertical technique is preferred when NAC elevation ranges from 2 to 4 cm and the base diameter of the contralateral breast requires some modification. Wise pattern mastopexy is considered when the degree of NAC elevation exceeds 4 cm and significant reshaping of the breast is required.

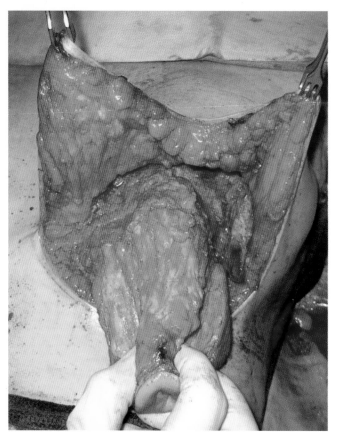

Figure 13.25 The inferior pedicle is created marinating the pectoral attachments and vascularity to improve vascularity of the NAC. The superior glandular resection has been completed.

Table 13.1 The classification for breast ptosis

Grade	Definition
1	NAC is at or slightly below the level of the IMF
2	NAC is below the level of the IMF
3	NAC is at the lowest position on the breast

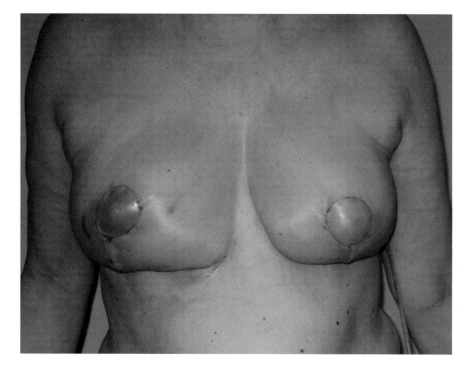

Figure 13.26 An early postoperative view demonstrating improved symmetry between the breasts with normal healing.

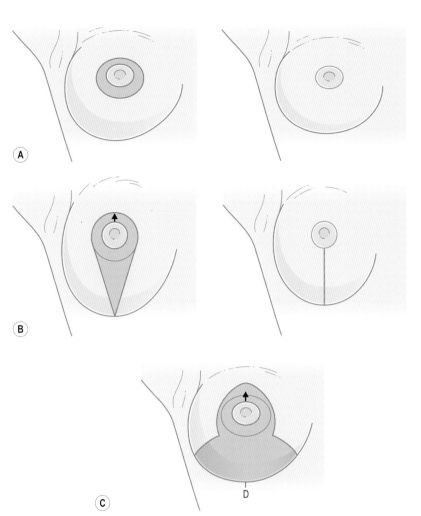

Figure 13.27 (**A**) Schematic illustration of the circumareolar approach to performing a mastopexy. (**B**) Schematic illustration of the circumvertical approach to performing a mastopexy. (**C**) Schematic illustration of a Wise pattern for mastopexy.

Markings and technique

The desired position of the NAC is delineated. This is usually based upon the location of the opposite NAC or the level of the IMF. For the circumareolar technique, an eccentric oval is delineated around the NAC, as depicted (**Fig. 13.28**). A crescent of non-areolar skin adjacent to the NAC is included within the marking. The areolar diameter may be reduced as desired but is usually set at 42 mm. The incisions are made around the NAC and around the delineated region. The crescent of skin is de-epithelialized. The dermis within the circumareolar pattern is scored and the breast parenchyma is partially undermined. This will promote easy mobilization of the NAC. The NAC is repositioned and the dermal edges are re-approximated with the perimeter dermis. An absorbable suture is generally preferred. The epidermis is reapproximated with a running subcuticular suture that can be absorbable or non-absorbable.

The circumvertical method is performed in a different fashion. Preoperative markings include the sternal midline, the breast meridian, and the IMF. The ideal location of the NAC is determined as previously described. A mosque type pattern is delineated, with the upper perimeter based at the superior aspect of the repositioned NAC.

The length of the mosque pattern ranges from 14 to 16 cm. The vertical limbs of the pattern are located below the level of the NAC. The medial and lateral vertical limbs are determined based on the degree of medial and lateral breast excursion. The inferior apex of the vertical limbs approaches the IMF. The delineated pattern and the NAC are incised. The dermal edges are scored and the parenchyma is partially undermined. Once complete, the NAC is repositioned within the mosque pattern and the dermal edges of the circumvertical design are reapproximated. The closure around the NAC is as previously described; however, the closure of the vertical limbs deserves mention. Often, the length of this limb is too long, resulting in an increase in the nipple to IMF distance. This is because the NAC has been elevated. Therefore, it is necessary to reduce the length of the incision. This is best accomplished using a subcuticular suture that is pulled tighter in order to reduce the length of the incision. This often results in a pleated appearance that will resolve over time. If this is not sufficient, then a small horizontal excision of skin and fat from the IMF is useful to decrease the length of the incision.

The inverted T or Wise pattern is occasionally used in women with significant ptosis. As with the two previous techniques, the ideal position of the NAC is determined

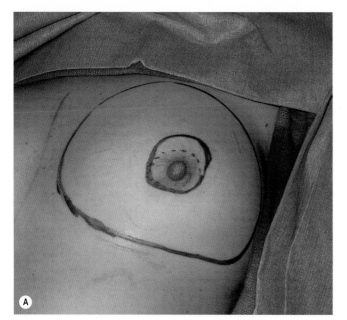

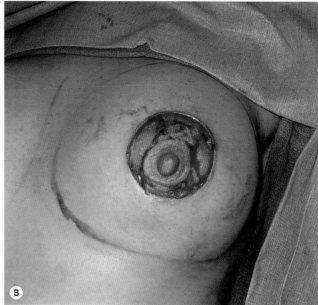

Figure 13.28 (**A**) The markings for a circumareolar mastopexy in a contralateral breast are illustrated. The elevated distance measures 1.5 cm. (**B**) The upper crescent of skin has been de-epithelialized and the dermal edges and superficial parenchyma have been scored. (**C**) The NAC is inset using absorbable sutures.

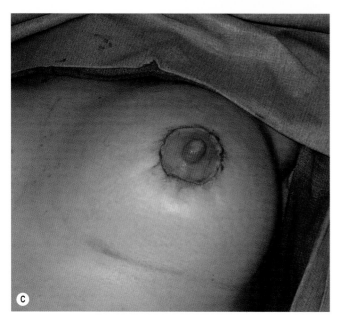

and the breast meridian and IMF are delineated. The markings for the Wise pattern are essentially the same as previously described for the breast reduction. The main difference is that the lengths of the vertical limbs of the pattern are usually 9–10 cm rather than 8 cm. In addition, all attempts are made to minimize the length of the horizontal incision and thus minimize the postoperative scarring. As with the other techniques, the pattern and the NAC are incised, the skin within the pattern is de-epithelialized, the dermal edges are scored, and the breast parenchyma is partially undermined. The degree of under-mining is usually more than previously described and often extends to the chest wall in order to mobilize the tissues without creating excessive distortion. The dermal edges are reapproximated using absorbable sutures. On

occasion, there may be excess fullness laterally and medially along the horizontal incision and some breast tissue may need to be removed. This maneuver will usually improve the shape and contour and result in a better outcome.

Contralateral augmentation following breast conservation or oncoplastic surgery

Contralateral breast augmentation is probably the least commonly performed operation on the contralateral following BCT or oncoplastic surgery. The primary indication is in a woman with micromastia who desires enhancement of breast volume and contour. A bilateral operation is usually requested; however, a unilateral augmentation may sometimes be performed. This operation is performed only on a delayed basis and is not recommended for at least 2 years following the postoperative radiation therapy on the ipsilateral breast.

There are several important factors that the surgeon should consider prior to performing this operation. The first is that the ipsilateral breast has been partially excised and radiated and the contralateral breast has not. This may result in varying degrees of postoperative asymmetry. It is important to estimate the volume discrepancy and select appropriately sized implants. The second is patient selection. The quality of the skin, subcutaneous, and glandular tissue must be assessed. This is obviously less important for the contralateral breast but is very important if an ipsilateral augmentation is being considered. Radiated tissue will lose some of its elasticity and the breast may not contour as desired. Finally, women must be informed that ongoing screening and surveillance will be necessary. Large devices or devices that are not properly inserted may obscure the visualization of the breast parenchyma. This may be a factor during mammography but will be less of an issue with an MRI scan.

Determining whether or not a woman is a candidate for implant surgery is important. As for all breast augmentation procedures, a clear understanding of motivations and expectations is required. In the rare case in which the contralateral breast is smaller than the cancerous breast, a contralateral augmentation may be performed. However, in women who desire bilateral augmentation special considerations are noted. In general, women who are considered at higher risk for recurrent or contralateral breast cancer should be cautioned about this procedure. However, women with stage 0 or 1 breast cancer who have not exhibited adverse sequelae to the radiation and have not had a recurrence can be considered for a bilateral operation. In all cases, it is recom-

mended that the surgical and medical oncologists concur with the desires of the patient and provide preoperative clearance. An example of a woman following bilateral breast augmentation following breast conservation therapy is shown (**Fig. 13.29**).

Optimizing outcomes

It is well appreciated that excellent outcomes are achieved more often when patient selection and surgical techniques have been optimized. In order to achieve excellent outcomes, several factors should be considered (**Box 13.2**). It is always important to assess patient expectations prior to commencing a surgical treatment plan. Women should understand that there may be complications or reasons to perform secondary procedures. All attempts will be made to achieve symmetry with a single procedure but only when this is deemed to be safe and in the best interests of the patient. Another factor is to appreciate the effects of radiation therapy. Although the ipsilateral breast is radiated, the effects will impact the outcome of a contralateral symmetry procedure. When a contralateral reduction mammaplasty is planned, it is recommended to reduce the contralateral breast slightly less to account for the postradiation shrinkage of the ipsilateral breast. Because of this phenomenon, a contralateral mastopexy

Box 13.2
Assess patient expectations
Delay contralateral procedures when tumor excision margins are uncertain
Perform contralateral augmentation or mastopexy on a delayed basis
Perform contralateral reduction mammoplasty on an immediate or delayed basis
Minimize scar length whenever possible

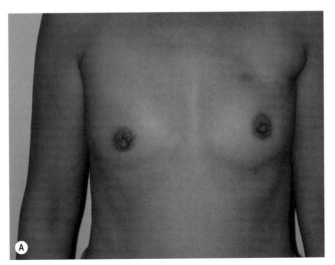
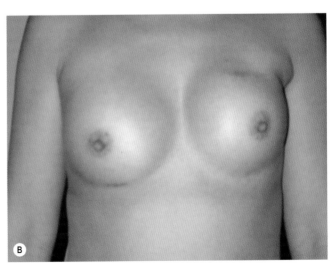

Figure 13.29 (**A**) Preoperative photograph of a woman who 3 years prior had a left lumpectomy and postoperative irradiation is shown. The plan is to perform a bilateral augmentation mammaplasty. (**B**) Postoperative photograph 2 years following breast augmentation with 150 cm³ saline breast implants is shown.

or augmentation should only be performed on a delayed basis after the postoperative changes have been identified. A subpectoral augmentation is preferable to a subglandular augmentation for the purposes of mammography and screening.

Complications and side effects

Reduction mammaplasty

Morbidities following breast reduction can occur but are minimized with proper patient selection and attention to operative details. The most common complications include but are not limited to bleeding, infection, complex scar, fat necrosis, loss of nipple–areolar sensation, delayed healing, inability to nurse, and persistent breast asymmetry. It is unrealistic to believe that complications following breast reduction can be completely avoided; however, they can be minimized. It is important to carefully assess the location of the NAC on both breasts. The vascularity of the NAC should be determined based on the presence of arterial and venous bleeding from the edges of the pedicle. When absent, a free nipple graft should be performed. On occasion, partial nipple necrosis may occur (**Fig. 13.30**). Hypertrophic scars are not common but often require revision when they occur (**Fig. 13.31**). Although there is no technique that will guarantee sensation of the NAC, studies have demonstrated that medial and inferior based pedicles achieve this more frequently.[25] Prevention of a hematoma requires meticulous hemostasis. When present, a hematoma may be identified by the use of postoperative drains. When used, drains are usually removed after 24 hours. Delayed healing is

usually the result of poor vascularity or excessive tension on the skin edges. It is important to design the reduction pattern so that excess tension on the skin edges does not occur. When it does occur, it is most often observed at the trifurcation point of the Wise pattern along the inframammary fold (**Fig. 13.32**).

Mastopexy

Mastopexy can result in many of the same morbidities that are observed following reduction mammaplasty. The most common, however, are related to the position and viability of the NAC as well as distortions in the cutaneous envelope. When performing a mastopexy, it is often recommended to decide upon the position of the NAC and assess the amount of skin to be excised. A technique that is generally regarded as safe is to use the 'tailor-tack' approach prior to excision of the skin. This will usually ensure that undue tension will not be a problem. In addition, the surgeon can assess breast contour. When the skin incisions are made, it is generally recommended to partially undermine the skin and superficial parenchyma in order to allow better mobilization of the skin flaps. This will usually result in less distortion.

Augmentation

Breast augmentation is complicated by the fact that no prosthetic device will last forever. Most devices will eventually fail over the course of one's lifetime. The most significant complications include capsular contracture, rupture, progressive distortion, asymmetry, and premature removal. Other considerations include compromised surveillance and patient dissatisfaction. Capsular contracture has been correlated with time. The longer a device

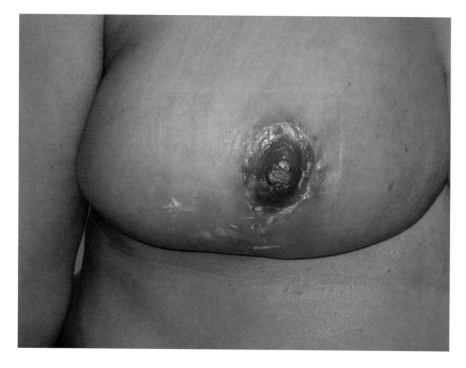

Figure 13.30 Delayed healing of the NAC following reduction mammaplasty.

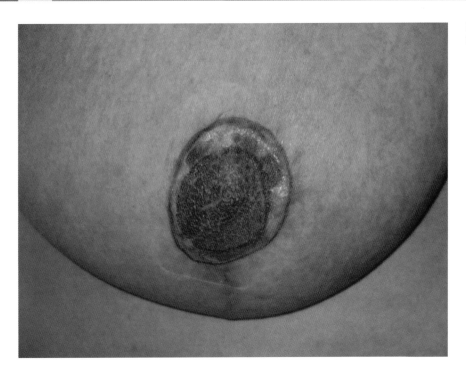

Figure 13.31 Hypertrophic scarring of the NAC following reduction mammaplasty.

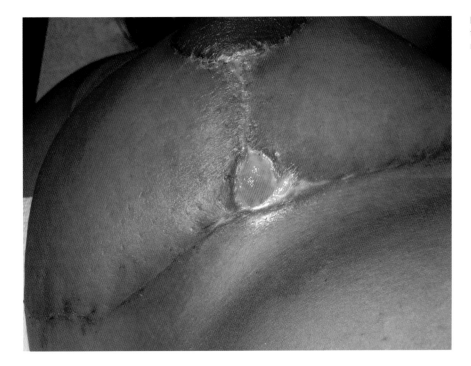

Figure 13.32 Delayed healing at the trifurcation point following reduction mammaplasty.

has been in place (usually greater than 10 years) the more likely it is to occur. Measures to minimize its occurrence in the short term include ensuring meticulous operative hemostasis, meticulous sterile technique, copious antibiotic irrigation, and use of antibiotics. With the current devices, failure is less common than previously reported, with a current incidence of 10% by 10 years. Rupture with saline devices is associated with rapid deflation; however, with silicone gel devices the rupture may be more difficult

to detect. MRI scans are recommended every few years to assess.

The issue of breast surveillance is important. It has been shown that the presence of a breast implant can obscure mammographic imaging of the breast in 30% of cases.[26] MRI scans may be the imaging study of choice in these cases. Placement of the implant in the subpectoral position may result in better imaging of the breast as the parenchymal–pectoral interface is not obscured by the implant.

Postoperative care

The postoperative care following contralateral breast surgery is the final consideration. In general, patients are instructed on how to care for the drains and what activities are appropriate. Women are instructed to shower on postoperative day 2 or 3. Antibiotics are prescribed for 5–7 days. Strenuous activities such as jogging, heavy lifting or other activities that entail some degree of bouncing are discouraged for 6 weeks. Women are instructed to wear a mildly supportive bra for 1 month. Mammograms are recommended no later than 6 months following the operation to determine the new baseline appearance of the breast. **Figure 13.33** illustrates the typical appearance of a mammogram following a reduction mammaplasty. **Figure 13.34** illustrates the appearance of fat necrosis following reduction mammaplasty.

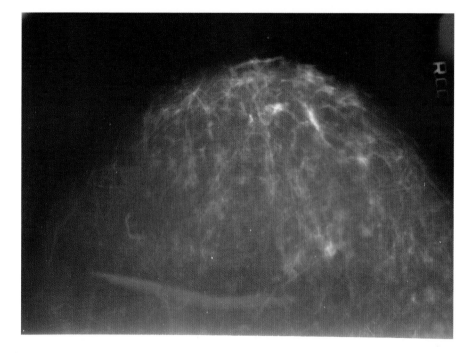

Figure 13.33 Normal mammogram following reduction mammaplasty.

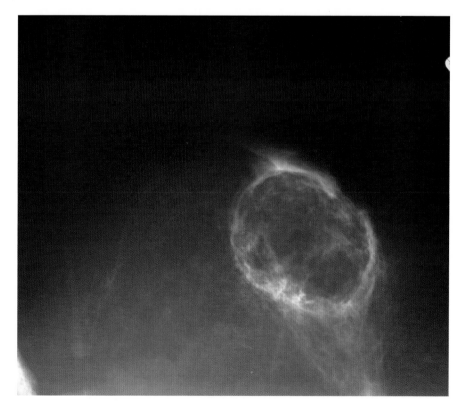

Figure 13.34 Fat necrosis following reduction mammaplasty.

Conclusions

Oncoplastic breast surgery is a safe alternative to mastectomy for some breast cancer patients. Although this management approach is designed to minimize breast disfigurement, it often results in considerable asymmetry between the breasts. This asymmetry can be successfully managed by employing a variety of techniques that are commonly used in cosmetic and reconstructive breast surgery. Proper patient selection and operative technique selection can provide excellent cosmetic outcomes and high patient satisfaction without compromising cancer detection.

References

1. Guyomard V, Leinster S, Wilkinson M. Systematic review of studies of patients' satisfaction with breast reconstruction after mastectomy. Breast 2007; 16:547–567.
2. Nahabedian MY. Symmetrical breast reconstruction: analysis of secondary procedures following reconstruction with implants and with autologous tissue. Plast Reconstr Surg 2005; 115:257–260.
3. Losken A, Carlson GW, Bostwick J, et al. Trends in unilateral breast reconstruction and the management of the contralateral breast. Plast Reconstr Surg 2002; 110:89–97.
4. Robbins GF, Berg JW. Bilateral primary breast cancers: a prospective clinicopathological study. Cancer 1964; 17:1501–1527.
5. Fisher F, Fisher B, Sass R, et al. Pathologic findings from the National Surgical Adjuvant Breast Project (protocol no. 4). Cancer 1984; 54:3002–3011.
6. Raabe W, Sauer T, Erichsen A, et al. Breast cancer in the contralateral breast: incidence and histopathology after unilateral radical treatment of the first breast cancer. Oncol Rep 1999; 6:1001–1007.
7. Kroll SS, Miller MJ, Schusterman MA, et al. Rationale for elective contralateral mastectomy with immediate breast reconstruction. Ann Surg Oncol 1994; 1:457–461.
8. Cook LS, White E, Schwartz SM, et al. A population-based study of contralateral breast cancer following a first primary breast cancer. Cancer Causes Control 1996; 7:382–390.
9. Heaton KM, Peoples GE, Singletary SE, et al. Feasibility of breast conservation therapy in metachronous or synchronous bilateral breast cancer. Ann Surg Oncol 1999; 6:102–108.
10. Healy EA, Cook EF, Orav EJ, et al. Contralateral breast cancer: clinical characteristics and impact on prognosis. J Clin Oncol 1993; 11:1545–1552.
11. Mariani L, Coradini D, Biganzoli E, et al. Prognostic factors for metachronous contralateral breast cancer: a comparison of the linear Cox regression model and its artificial neural network extension. Breast Cancer Res Treat 1997; 44:167–178.
12. Singletary EE, Taylor SH, Guinee VF, et al. Occurrence and prognosis of contralateral carcinoma of the breast. J Am Coll Surg 1994; 178:390–396.
13. Roubidoux MA, Helvie MA, Wilson TE, et al. Women with breast cancer: histologic findings in the contralateral breast. Radiology 1997; 203:691–694.
14. Losken A, Elwood ET, Styblo TM, et al. The role of reduction mammaplasty in reconstructing partial mastectomy defects. Plast Reconstr Surg 2002; 109:968–975.
15. Spear SL, Pelletiere CV, Wolfe AJ, et al. Experience with reduction mammaplasty combined with breast conservation therapy in the treatment of breast cancer. Plast Reconstr Surg 2003; 111:1102–1109.
16. Clough KB, Thomas SS, Fitoussi AD, et al. Reconstruction after conservative treatment for breast cancer: cosmetic sequelae classification revisited. Plast Reconstr Surg 2004; 114:1743–1753.
17. Ecklund GW, Busby RC, Miller SH, et al. Improved imaging of the augmented breast. Am J Roentgenol 1988; 151:469–473.
18. Palmer JH, Taylor GI. The vascular territories of the anterior chest wall. Br J Plast Surg 1986; 39:287–299.
19. Jaspars JJP, Posma AN, van Immerseel AAH, et al. The cutaneous innervation of the female breast and nipple–areola complex: implications for surgery. Br J Plast Surg 1997; 50:249–259.
20. Nahabedian MY, McGibbon BM, Manson PN. Medial pedicle reduction mammaplasty for severe mammary hypertrophy. Plast Reconstr Surg 2000; 105:896–904.
21. Mofid MM, Dellon AL, Elias JJ, et al. Quantitation of breast sensibility following reduction mammaplasty: a comparison of inferior and medial pedicle techniques. Plast Reconstr Surg 2002; 109:2283–2288.
22. Nahabedian MY, Mofid M. Viability and sensation of the nipple areolar complex following reduction mammaplasty. Ann Plast Surg 2002; 49:24–32.
23. Mofid MM, Klatsky SA, Singh NK, et al. Nipple–areola complex sensitivity after primary breast augmentation: a comparison of peri-areolar and inframammary incision approaches. Plast Reconstr Surg 2006; 117:1694–1698.
24. Nahabedian MY, Galdino G. Symmetric breast reconstruction: is there a role for three-dimensional digital photography? Plast Reconstr Surg 2003; 112:1582–1590.
25. Schlenz I, Rigel S, Schemper M, et al. Alteration of nipple areolar sensitivity by reduction mammaplasty: a comparison of five techniques. Plast Reconstr Surg 2005; 115:743–751.
26. Handel N, Silverstein M. Breast cancer diagnosis and prognosis in augmented women. Plast Reconstr Surg 2006; 118:587–593.

Index